1500 Affirmations for Black Women

5-books-in-1 to transform your life with money, power, inner peace, health, family and dreams

Ola Diallo

© Copyright 2022 Intuitive Way Publishing. All rights reserved.

The content contained within this book may not be reproduced, duplicated or transmitted without direct written permission from the author or the publisher. Under no circumstances will any blame or legal responsibility be held against the publisher, or author, for any damages, reparation, or monetary loss due to the information contained within this book, either directly or indirectly.

Legal Notice:

This book is copyright protected. It is only for personal use. You cannot amend, distribute, sell, use, quote or paraphrase any part, or the content within this book, without the consent of the author or publisher.

Disclaimer Notice:

Please note the information contained within this document is for educational and entertainment purposes only. All effort has been executed to present accurate, up to date, reliable, complete information. No warranties of any kind are declared or implied. Readers acknowledge that the author is not engaged in the rendering of legal, financial, medical or professional advice. The content within this book has been derived from various sources. Please consult a licensed professional before attempting any techniques outlined in this book.

By reading this document, the reader agrees that under no circumstances is the author responsible for any losses, direct or indirect, that are incurred as a result of the use of the information contained within this document, including, but not limited to, errors, omissions, or inaccuracies.

Editor: Nigel Lavers
Intuitive Way Publishing is a division of Hedhaus Inc
158F Brairwynd Court, Edmonton, AB, Canada, T5T OH4
ISBN: 9798832549422
Cover art: 99designs
www.intuitive-way.com

Table of Contents

REAP WEALTH, CREATE HEALTH, AND PASSIONATELY LOVE WITH THE POWER OF YOUR WORDS 1

- INTRODUCTION 3
  - *Goals* 5
  - *Start* 6
  - *Authenticity* 7
- CHAPTER 1: AFFIRMATIONS TO WARM UP THE SOUL, *WITH MONEY* 9
  - *Money* 12
- CHAPTER 2: AFFIRMATIONS TO PROTECT YOURSELF, *WITH HEALING ENERGY* 21
- CHAPTER 3: AFFIRMATIONS OF SELF-LOVE, *FOR BLACK WOMEN* 33
- CONCLUSION 46

POWERFUL MANIFESTATIONS TO REALIZE THE WISDOM OF FORGIVENESS AND YOUR DIVINE FEMININE 49

- INTRODUCTION 51
  - *Goals* 58
- CHAPTER 4: AFFIRMATIONS TO ACCEPT PEACE AND STAND POWERFUL 60
- CHAPTER 5: AFFIRMATIONS TO EMBRACE SELF-LOVE AND TO FIND JUSTICE IN FORGIVENESS 74
- CHAPTER 6: AFFIRMATIONS TO UNEARTH THE DIVINE FEMININE WITHIN ME, BECAUSE WE KNOW WE ARE POWERFUL BLACK WOMEN 87
- CONCLUSION 97

REMEMBER YOUR INNER CHILD, PERFECT YOUR SELF-IMAGE, AND IGNITE THE FIRE OF SEX 99

- INTRODUCTION 101
- CHAPTER 7: AFFIRMATIONS TO REMEMBER YOUR INNER CHILD 105
- CHAPTER 8: AFFIRMATIONS TO PERFECT YOUR SELF-IMAGE 122
- CHAPTER 9: AFFIRMATIONS TO IGNITE THE POWER OF SEX 135

Conclusion 145

WELCOME THE NATURE OF MOTHERS, NURTURE THE INNOCENCE OF DAUGHTERS, AND MANIFEST THE CAREER OF YOUR DREAMS 147

Introduction 149
Chapter 10: Affirmations to Welcome the Nature of Mothers
.... 153
Chapter 11: Affirmations to Nurture the Innocence of Daughters 164
Chapter 12: Affirmations to Manifest the Career of Your Dreams 174
   Affirmations When Looking For Work 183
   Affirmations for the Big Interview 184
   Affirmations for Your First Day at Work 187
   Affirmations to Keep You Motivated 188
   Affirmations to Succeed at Your Career 189
Conclusion 191

DROP THE EXCUSES—DREAM BIG, THINK POSITIVELY, LIVE A LIFE OF ACCOMPLISHMENT AND ACHIEVEMENT 195

Introduction 197
   Goals 200
Chapter 13: Drop the Excuses—Dream Big 203
Chapter 14: Think Positively 215
Chapter 15: Live a Life of Accomplishment and Achievement 224
Conclusion 234
References 239
   Image References 245

— For my daughters,

my husband,

my parents

and me,

the small black child

who I remember all too fondly —

Reap Wealth, Create Health, And Passionately Love With The Power Of Your Words

Introduction

Affirmations invoke the power of the verb. The verb is the most evocative and irreplaceably creative spell that we may ever cast. Love may be the creative force, emblematic of fire and passion. But our voice is miraculous. As we comprehend ourselves and awaken to the powers within, we manifest our destinies. I awaken my subconscious by using the spoken word and putting it into action. This is like striking a gong–it puts our consciousness into activity. By way of positive thinking and acting through our fears, we can conquer our desires and achieve ultimate fulfillment, today and every day.

This book aims to give you the option of merely reading, yes, but also learning to speak with true power! Gain your deepest sense of self by believing the words you read, and also speaking them. Use what I am writing for your benefit–find a deep aha! as you remark in your ability to project your imagination onto the screen of your mind with your words. Let your clairaudient senses awaken to clairvoyance! In this book I have affirmations to offer you as practices which will develop your skills in speaking with authenticity, acting as your true self, and knowing your inner child is protected and revered for its immaculate nature.

Black women deal with elements which are unique to them. For the black women of our youth these elements force them to mature quite quickly and in unique ways. We should be mindful of racism, sexism, and various obvious stressors and prejudices which exist within western society. With all of this burden, which we have grown up in, this unique book of affirmations was created.

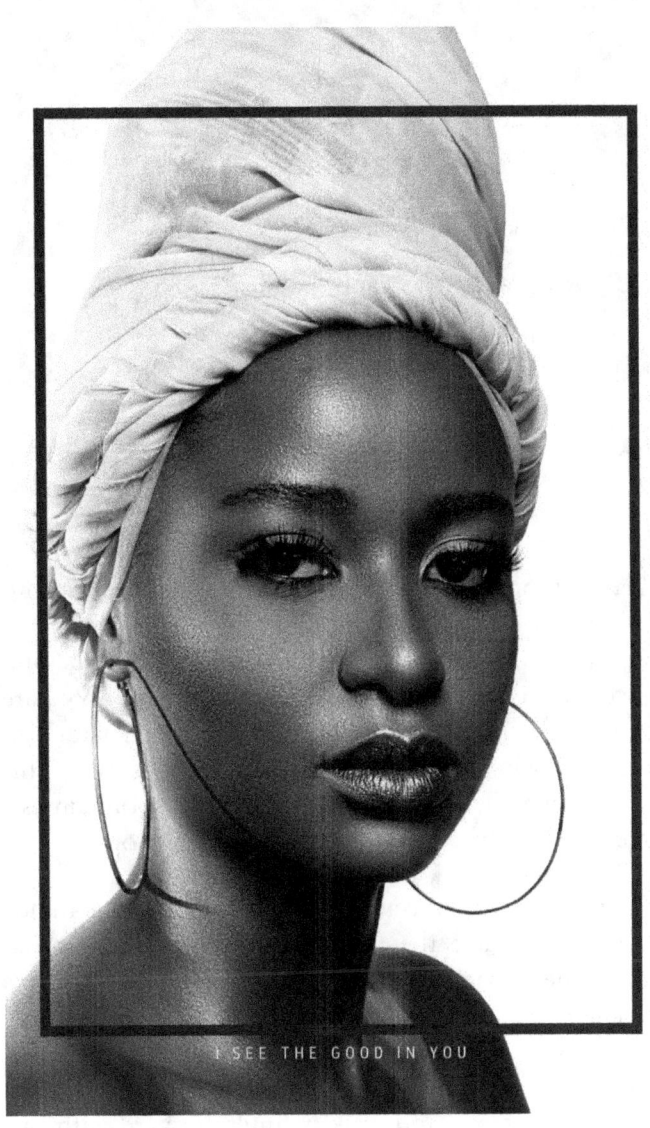

I SEE THE GOOD IN YOU

Goals

The goals of this book are threefold, and simple:
1. Awaken our desires,
2. Crystalize our resolve, and
3. Manifest our destiny.

Start

What's stopping us from manifesting our desires into reality? We don't know the formula! If there is such a formula at all? I try to eradicate bad habits and subconscious behaviors... It isn't easy! We are sometimes stricken with foul moods, ridden with bad luck, or stuck with impossible problems to solve. This is what generally troubles many among us. Sometimes I have even felt triggered to give up and lose hope.

We are going to start at the beginning. Let our minds be at ease–I have the formula! It is going to unfold within these pages. We can feel reassured that this book is a very powerful source of creative energy which will ultimately reach our hearts—by using our voice. In fact, we are going to unlock our hidden potential, dissolve our fears, and walk mightily forward with our family and peers by our side.

Authenticity

Learning to live with passion, to aspire to accomplish our dreams, and to discover our destiny is a universal axiom. So, if everyone knows this, how come so few are reaching it? The answer is in authenticity. Learning to be authentic is of course a unique and grand task. For example, rarely does a grandmaster find a pupil capable of handling the mighty teachings of manifestation–but here, we are about to prove to ourselves that we have the ability to crystalize our self-image by reframing our thoughts. We want to know our capabilities are limitless, and that the life we desire can be reached. Here is the method of thinking, feeling, moving to do just that. To triumph and take advantage of these positive statements, we will have to live through these words as they become ours. I do not reserve them just for me—I share them now. By reformatting our thinking pathways, we will achieve breakthroughs in our personal and private lives. As we practice these affirmations, we may become confronted with the feelings of fulfilling them with action! It is with courage we take this plunge everyday–and we become authentic in as a result. We mean what we say when we see ourselves achieving and acting through these affirmations. We will become who we see ourselves as–simply put. Our self-image is manufactured through our words, enjoyed through our actions, and realized through our deeds. Let's be careful though, taking worthless actions without a personal sense of integrity will only last so long. Lying to ourselves about who we truly are inevitably ends in failure or regret. And starving ourselves from taking a risk never gets us anywhere. Narrow is the way through—the intuitive way.

So starting now, with our words made flesh we are becoming vibrations of cosmic authority. Our heartbeat, brain rhythms, and vocal vibrations are about to unite into harmony, octave after octave, until we reach climax after climax of complete self-realization.

We are going to realize these affirmations of manifestation with the use of crystal gemstones as well as the word of the Holy Bible. Crystals help to tune our vibrations with their amazing properties of atomic structure. By keeping these recommended crystals with us as we practice these affirmations, we are harnessing our intention to the measurable effects of the majesty of the Earth. We can keep these recommended stones in our car while we listen to audio, in our lap while we read, or at our bedside while we vocalize these affirmations the first moment we awake!

Finding novelty in our affirmations is important to be playful–this is a lighthearted affair between our connection with God and ourselves, with truly mighty results on the other side of practice.

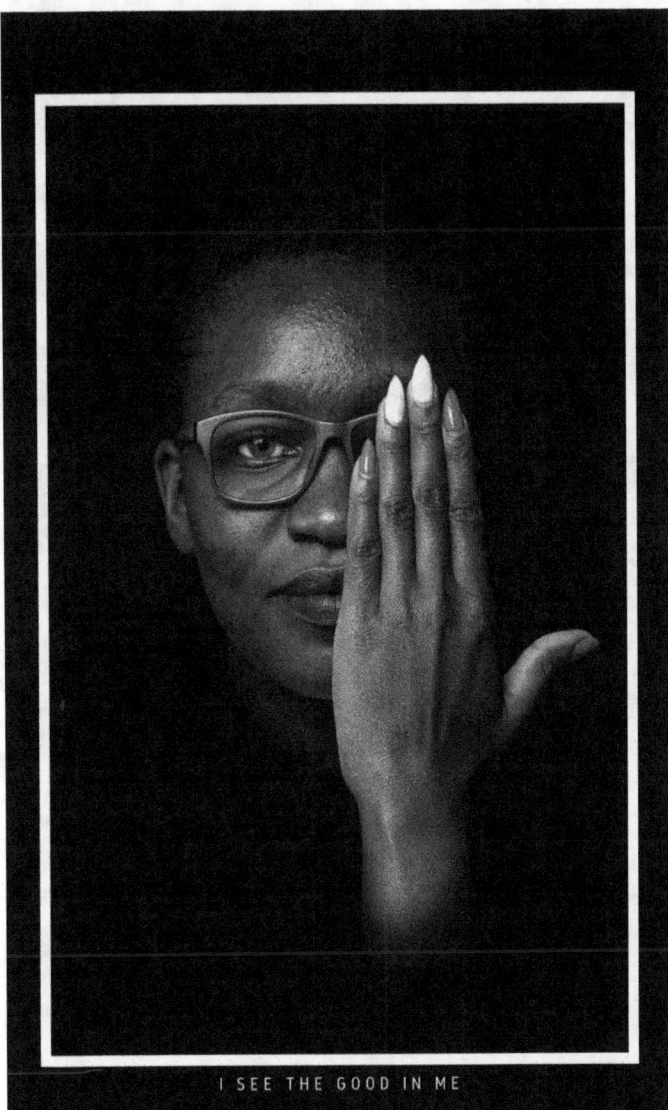

Chapter 1:

Affirmations to Warm up the Soul, *with money*

The recommended crystals for this chapter's series of affirmations are Jade, Malachite, and Garnet. All three of these crystals, when combined in unison, are going to promote attitudes of bliss with respect to money. I start with money as the first topic, with a warm-up to manifestation in general. Money is often the most difficult subject to analyze between friends and family when it comes to our personal and private life. Finding harmony with money in our daily life is like releasing ourselves from the idea of sin! Comon! Life is meant to be enjoyed; so, let's manage our attitudes with respect to money before we move onto other exciting avenues of our life experience.

"Whoever gathers money

little by little makes it grow."

—Proverbs 13:11

For those listening, follow the prompts. If you are reading, remember to repeat this not just mentally, but with your voice. You can do it girl, this is a profound change! The world is waiting and you have the power! Use your voice, and believe in what makes you ultimately powerful—your voice and your projections of fire! Into the mirror, as you drive, while riding your bike, through mountainous terrain, as you put on your makeup, especially in the shower or in front of the mirror! Look girl I believe in you, your destiny is yours and yours only. Find it within yourself, use your words, and repeat these now.

I allow my dreams to become reality

I attract into my life all the things that I want

I am manifesting the future I want, right now

I am magnetic for dreams and goals

I am achieving my dreams

I live in a wonderful loving house in a lovely neighborhood

I am a good thing and good things happen every day in my life

I enjoy being successful in every way

I have an abundance of love and happiness in my life

I enjoy healthy and a life full of positive energy

Money

New amounts of money are coming into my life

I manifest money more and more every day

I live with financial abundance

I enjoy wealth and prosperity in my life

I am an abundant ocean of wealth

Wealth pours into my bank account like waves on a shore

I am open to wealth and prosperity

I live a prosperous, wealthy life

My business enjoys paying customers

There is enough money in the Universe for everyone and there is enough money for me

I am constantly attracting money into my life

The energies that create abundance are in harmony with my mind

I am watching money making opportunities come into my life

Every day, I get more and more comfortable with having a lot of money

I am feeling happy with accruing a lot of wealth

The Universe is delivering to me all the money I need, and more and more

I can achieve success, and others too

I greet my bank manager with a smile

Piles and piles of money are building up in my bank account

I am employed with a wonderful job and terrific salary

My finances are improving beyond my dreams

Paying customers want my business

My goals with money are being realized

Money is appearing in my life through many channels and harmonious ways

Having money feels good

I have the means to spend money on the things I want

I am fulfilling my money goals easily, day-by-day

Money loves me and keeps coming to me

I am financially successful

I am a leader in financial decisions

Wealth and money are comfortable topics in my life

I enjoy money and wealth as a part of my life

I am open to being beyond wealthy in my life

There is an abundance of wealth in my life

Money flows into my bank account like a river into the ocean

I have an excellent financial situation

I attract money to myself easily and effortlessly

I am a magnet for money

I release all inhibitions to being wealthy

I release resistance to attracting money

I release any traumas from loss I had from money

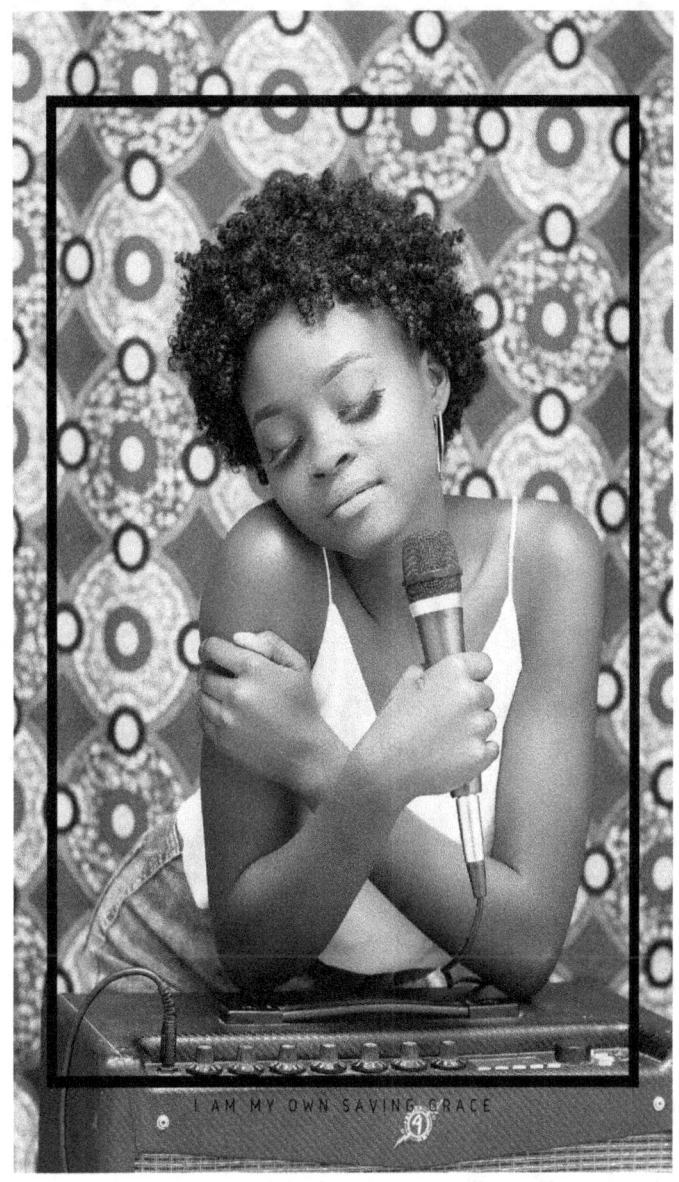

I accept and receive gifts of money and wealth

Money is attracted to me

Prosperity is alive in me

Money comes to me easily and effortlessly

Wealth flows into my life constantly

My finances are improving beyond my wildest dreams

Money is coming to me at this very moment

I remain open and receptive to a wealthy life

Money and happiness co-exist together in abundance

My wildest dreams of money are coming true

I am receiving money and I am open to more and more

When I focus on joy, I receive money

I attract money for myself and others

I have an abundance of money to share with others

I give and share money with those I love

Money is like energy, it flows into my life constantly

I am attuned to the flow of money, and I respect it

I hold the power to bring money into my life

I hold the power of attracting unlimited wealth

There is an abundance of money in my life, and I welcome more and more

I attract money in abundance for myself and others

My prosperity is unlimited and money also unlimited

I have money pouring into my life

My abundance of money is enriching my life

My mind is a powerful agent to handle money and wealth

I walk through the world free of concern for money

Money flows to me as I walk through the world

I will attain all the riches I wish for

I am on my way to attaining my independent wealth

I have everything I need to be wealthy and prosperous

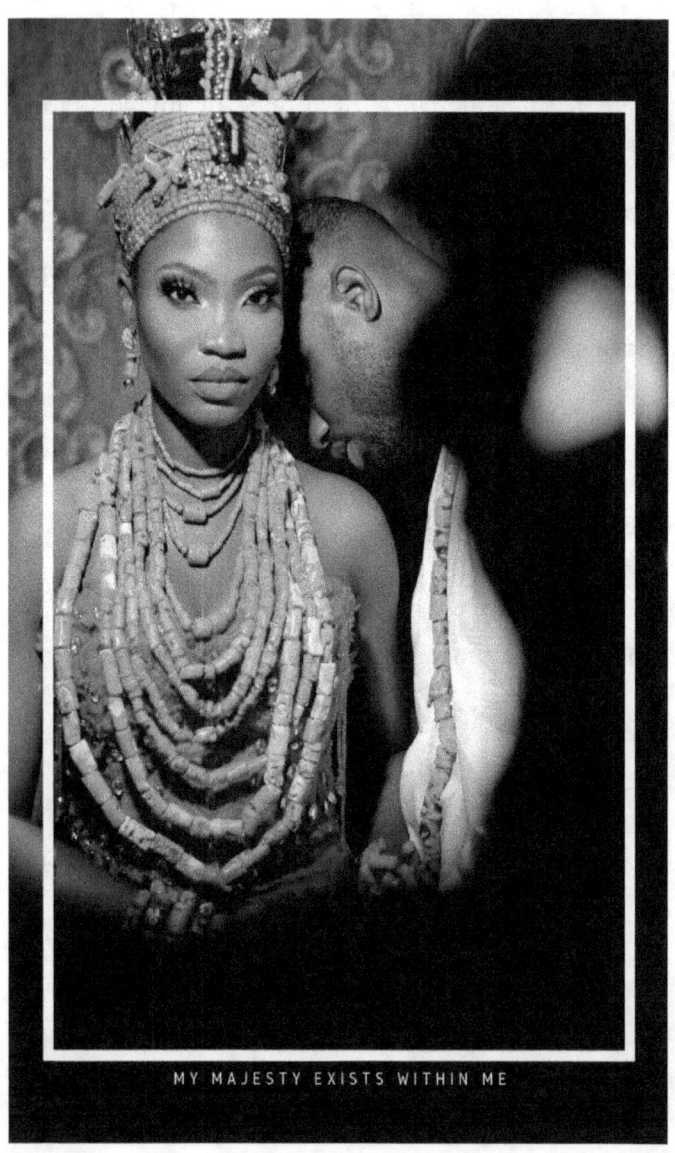

MY MAJESTY EXISTS WITHIN ME

There is money everywhere around me, I just need to take it

I attract money in every endeavor I undertake

I love attracting money

Money is a mystery, and I enjoy it falling into my lap

Money flows miraculously into my bank account

People love giving me money

I permit other to become wealthy with me

I am aligned with wealth and prosperity

The energy of wealth and abundance nourishes me

I allow money to flow freely to me

Money comes to me, in every monet

I am grateful that I can manifest money to my liking

By thinking this way, I am manifesting a present state of abundance

More and more, money is coming my way every minute

Money flows to me with ease and comfort

I focus on the flow of money and how it helps me

I see abundance all around me

Money chooses me–and I choose money

With these words, I visualize having money and receiving more money

Money finds its home with me, always

Money falls into place in my life

Wealth is attracted to me from every direction

Massive amounts of money are piling up for me

I breathe calmly and smell my money near me

Prosperity calms my soul and I breathe it in

I allow prosperity to energy my life

I am a master of money and wealth

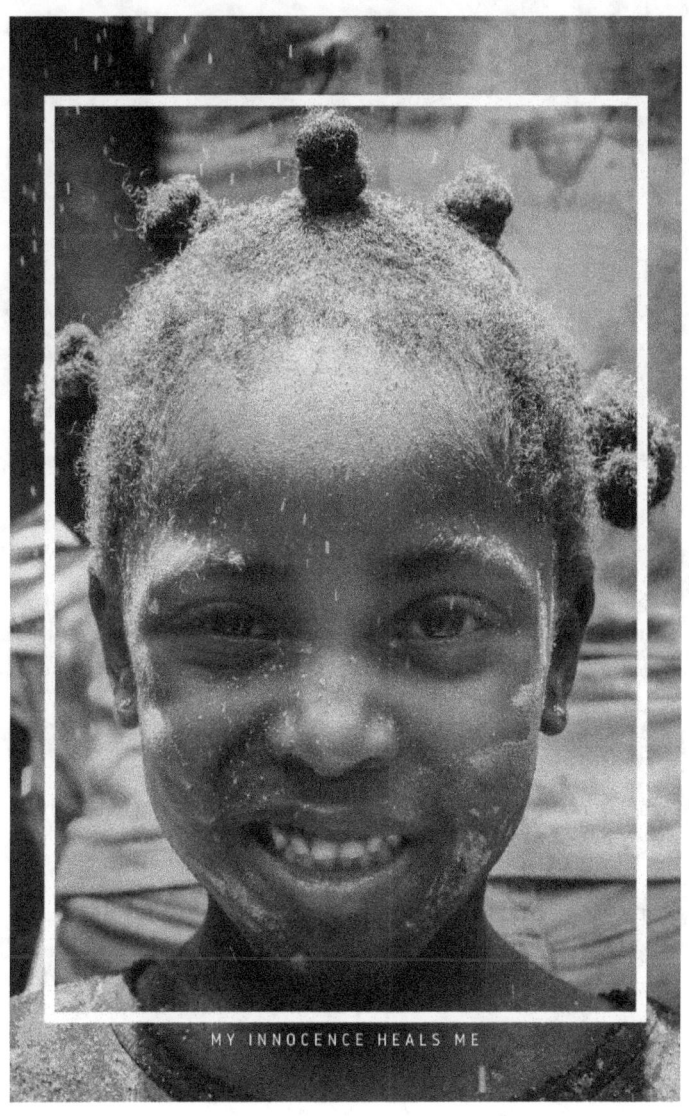

Chapter 2:

Affirmations to protect yourself, *with healing energy*

Again, the spoken word is powerful when confidence is found, and integrity is used. We should learn to follow through on our word. Also, we should learn to have courage with our actions, as they follow our words into actualizations, through to manifestation.

The joy of healing begins now, as we visualize ourselves enjoying the passions we so desire to complete.

Let's be prepared to lose our sense of doubt and dream big–let the changes occur in our life as we speak these words. These affirmations are found to manifest our destiny.

The changes will be subtle, but like the first words of a child, these changes will also be magnificent. Let's keep a childlike state of mind through this chapter and a sense of innocence will pervade.

Our healing energies will become intuitive, and our self-image will be transformed into one with an awakened sense of purpose.

The crystals recommended for this chapter are oh-so-great–**Clear Quartz, Carnelian, and Moldavite**. Of course, moldavite is hard to get, and has a vibration which is tough to handle, that's why we warmed up with a chapter on money. Rare stones are expensive, but when these incantations are performed well, we won't regret the choice of gemstone.

> *"My God, my rock, in whom I take refuge,*
>
> *my shield, and the horn of my salvation,*
>
> *my stronghold and my refuge,*
>
> *my savior; you save me"*
>
> *–2 Samuel 22:3*

It really is this simple. Let's begin.

I am alive and in good health

I choose good health with every thought of everyday

My health is important to me

Wealth is also health

My body and mind function in harmony

I radiate perfect health and vitality

Each day, I discover new ways to enjoy good health

I am deserving of a healthy mind, spirit, and body

I invest in my health with every decision I make

I am responsible for my health, and I promote healing as a model with others

I nurture myself with water and nutrients

I bless my water and food as sacred medicine for my soul

I respect my doctors as they treat my body and mind with medicine

I care for my body and mind with healthy eating

I choose foods that promote good thoughts, happy emotions, and feeling of joy

I feel myself and my family with vital nutrients

I enjoy cooking and eating healthy foods

I trust my body as the spiritual temple for adoration

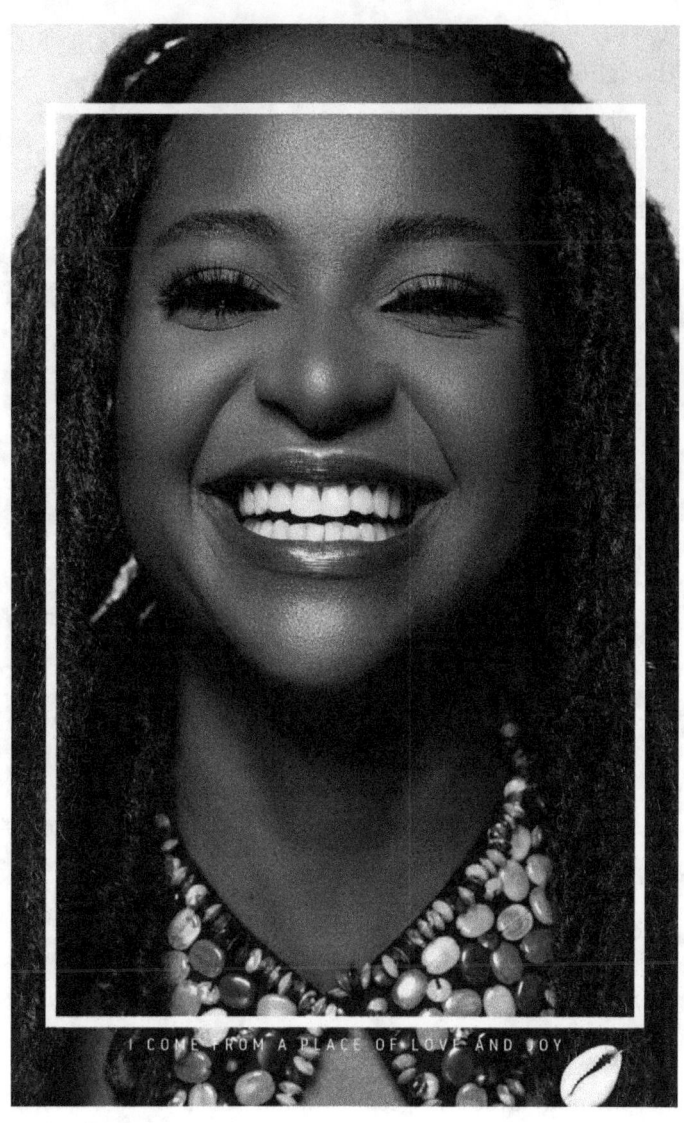

My body tells me what it needs, through emotions and thoughts that I observe

When I choose foods, I feel good eating them

I savor my time to eat as a sacred ritual of happiness

I use the energy of my body for fitness and strength

I stay healthy because I deserve to feel good everyday

I keep my body in tip-top shape

I feel grateful of my body functioning in harmony

I am overflowing with an abundance of energy

I care for my health as a gift of love has been given to me

I cherish my gifts of health and I nurture them with love and gratefulness

My fitness goals are uniquely mine and I own them as good habits

I act and behave in harmony with my body

I love how my body rushes with energy before and after I exercise

My immune system is healthy and robust

I praise my body for its ability to heal itself

My body heals when I sleep, heals when I eat, and heals when I care for it

My health gets better and better everyday

Healing is my passion

Healing is my perfection

Healing is my journey

I welcome feelings of healing energy

My illness and pain don't define me

I act to heal, and heal to act

I celebrate my healing journey with milestones and achievements

The wisdom of my intuition is a healing act

I am a brave and resilient healer

I cherish my healing journey for the wisdom I am earning

I do the best I can, and the best is good enough

I feel grateful for the health I have today

My healthy body, mind, and spirit are all beautifully harmonized

I am beautiful just as I am

I embrace my imperfections

I let myself age gracefully

My look is young and my life full of vigor and enthusiasm

I am happy being alive and living in good health

I am worthy of my healing journey

I am allowed to struggle and feel compassion for myself

I am allowed to find my voice

I am not alone in my healing journey

My past does not define me

I find wisdom in my experiences

I release blame from any trauma in my past

I am a forgiving person

I draw boundaries and protect my healthy

I deserve to have my own space

I understand that it's okay to be the way I am

I release myself from feelings of fear and indignation

I embrace my healthy habits with devotion

I feel safe and protected

My life is my own, no one has permission to say otherwise

My true ability lies in my love for myself and my love for others

My healing journey is not always sugarplums and buttercups

I respect myself in my healing journey despite bad days, weeks, or months

I release myself from judgment, and find innocence as I bounce back

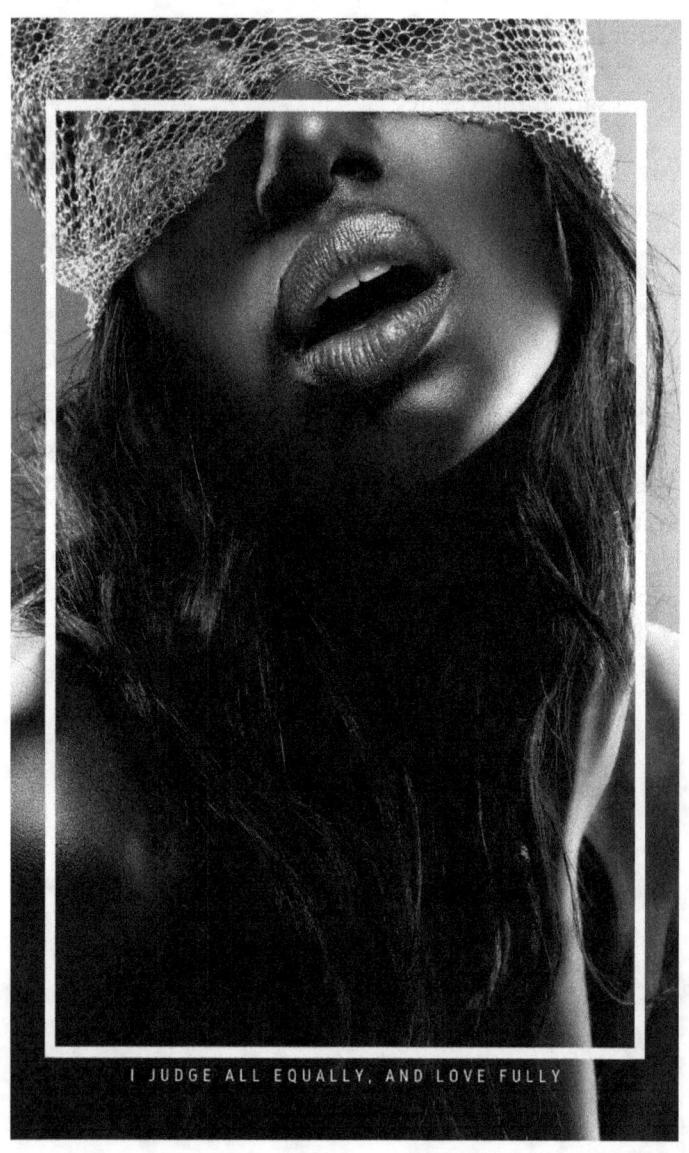

Every breathe of mine heals me

I am abiding in loving kindness

When I feel emotional, I acknowledge my feelings gracefully

It's okay to make mistakes, I forgive myself and I forgive others

I am a glorious pearl of magnificent value

The world will enjoy my presence

I am helpful to others, and I seek help for anything I need

I survived the worst and I'm prepared for the best

Life rewards me with happiness

I embrace change as I heal myself and better my life

I let myself feel and experience my emotions

I trust my gut instinct

My emotions are valid and my heart warms when I cherish my life

When I feel hurt, I seek care

Caring people love me

What I am afraid of does not limit me

I release all fears from letting me heal

I am a survivor and I live a complete life

I release judgment and express my individuality freely

Healing makes me feel better and I encourage others to heal too

I am patient and I heal in my own time

I am worthy of love and affection

I am worthy of a healing hand

I protect my emotional wounds like my physical ones

I nurture and protect myself

I become stronger as I venture forth into the world

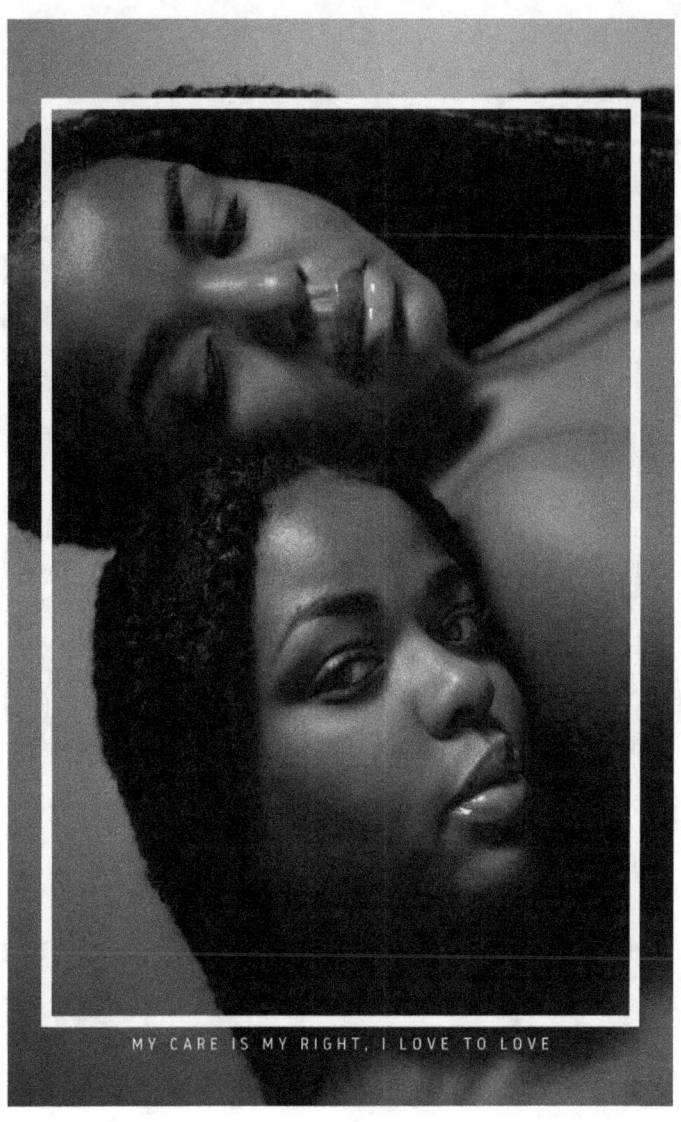

Chapter 3:

Affirmations of Self-Love, *for Black Women*

Special instructions: we should hold these stones in our hand or place them on our altar as we set our intentions through vocalizing these affirmations. Remember, these are affirmations of manifestation, and to manifest, we use our creative verb, our voice. So, finding a spot in private at home, in our car, or while on a walk is fine. Alternatively, you can vocalize and follow along with a group. Actually, a group is better, but we'll need to carry each other along while listening and speaking at the same time.

"Let us love one another,

for love comes from God.

Everyone who loves has been

born of God and knows God"

—John 4:7-21

One of these stones will work, or two, or the complete combination of all three—**Rose Quartz, Moonstone, and Rhodochrosite.**

We are all survivors in the world, yet survival is the most basic instinct we use when setting ourselves up for a future in which to *thrive* beyond just surviving. Don't get me wrong, as we become adjusted to enjoying surviving and thriving, we seek to step out of our comfort zone, and take on more and more experiences. Unless we take time for self-love, this act of expanding our comfort zone through adventure can leave us desperately stuck in the rat-race of Monday to Friday.

Enjoy these affirmations of manifestation for their aim to ignite fires of self-love inside our every day. As we manage them into our schedule, we'll slowly build and reinforce our instincts to better and better our daily experiences.

I accept myself as I am today

Right now, I am exactly as I need to be

I find unconditional love for myself

I accept love gracefully

I feel at peace with myself

I am at peace, while loving others

I am an abundant supply of love for myself and others

I embrace who I am

I am just as perfect as the day I was born

I create love with every breath I take

There is enough love for everyone to enjoy

I am growing, evolving, and becoming my best self

I am worthy of this time, to care for myself

My heart is filled light and love

My mind is shining bright with clarity

I laugh regularly and love to attend to my happiness

I enjoy spreading happiness and love with others

My needs matter to me and I prioritize them

I follow my heart, living my dreams

I am disciplined to set goals true to me and vision for myself

I deserve the life I want for myself

I love the person I am, and the person I am becoming

I earn my keep and protect those I love unconditionally

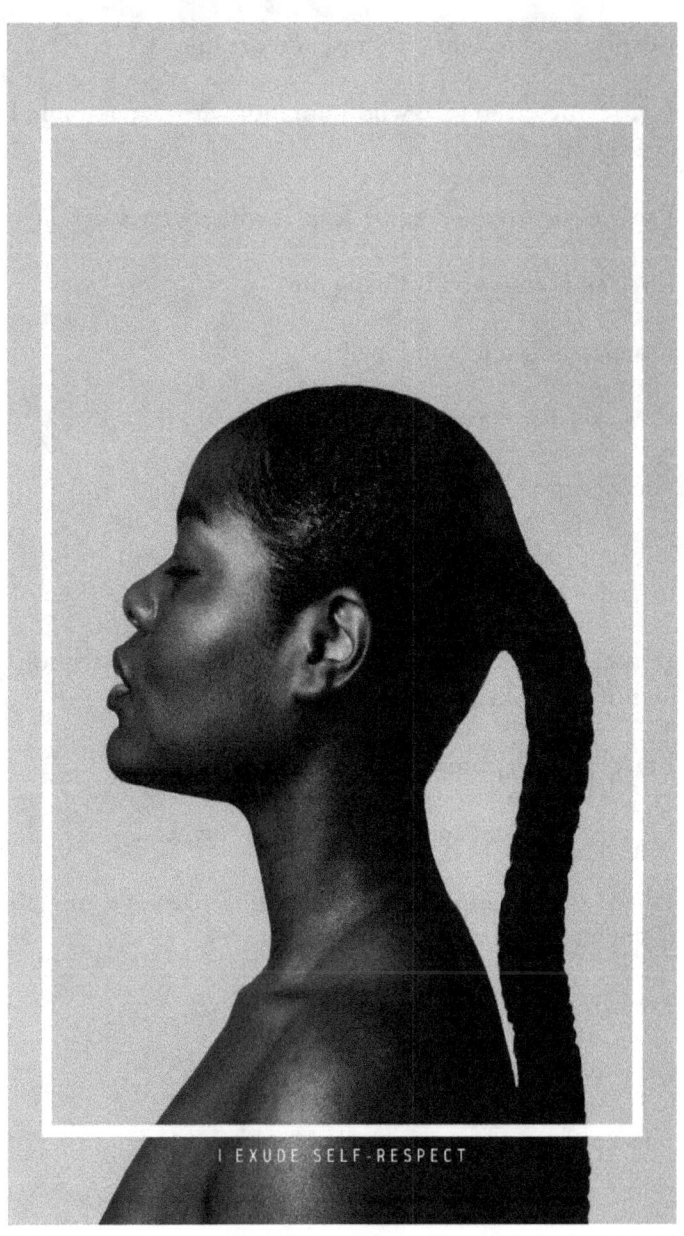

I express my feelings, desires, and dreams

I allow myself to love who I am, not who others thing I should be

I set boundaries and enjoy feeling authentic to myself

I live an honest and fulfilling life

I love myself unconditionally

I sow seeds of love by asking to help others

I accept myself when others want to help me

I accept judgment and criticism for its value in knowing myself

I accept that I have fears and doubts without identifying with them

I give myself approval to learn and grow

I accept my fears and doubts and try anyways

I am courageous and brave as I observe myself changing to better my life

I release myself from pain and suffering

I was born to love and be loved

I accept love, prosperity and abundance

I nurture myself with love and tenderness

I am grateful for this body, mind, and soul

I use my body, mind and soul to fulfill my destiny

I am a mighty, glorious person

My soul shines through the darkness

I have divine creative powers

My innocence is mine and I preserve it

I live my life for me and lead others to feel the same about themselves

I think positively about myself

I am capable of overcoming my imperfections

I am compassionate with myself when I fail

I overcome difficult challenges with patience and compassion

I release myself from anxiety and depression and find enthusiasm instead

I uplift spirits and forgive others who wronged me

I release those who judge with forgiveness and compassion

I wake every morning loving myself

I wake believing every day is going to be a great day

When I lay my head down at night I appreciate what my life is becoming

I am thrilled to live a life of fulfillment

I trust the knowledge of myself and I am at peace with myself

I cultivate habits to serve me and better my life

My love life is full of joy, pleasure and fun

I greet lovers with enthusiasm and an open heart

I enjoy sex for its pleasurable fulfilment

I greet my lover with words of care and commitment

I am deeply loved and I carry myself this way

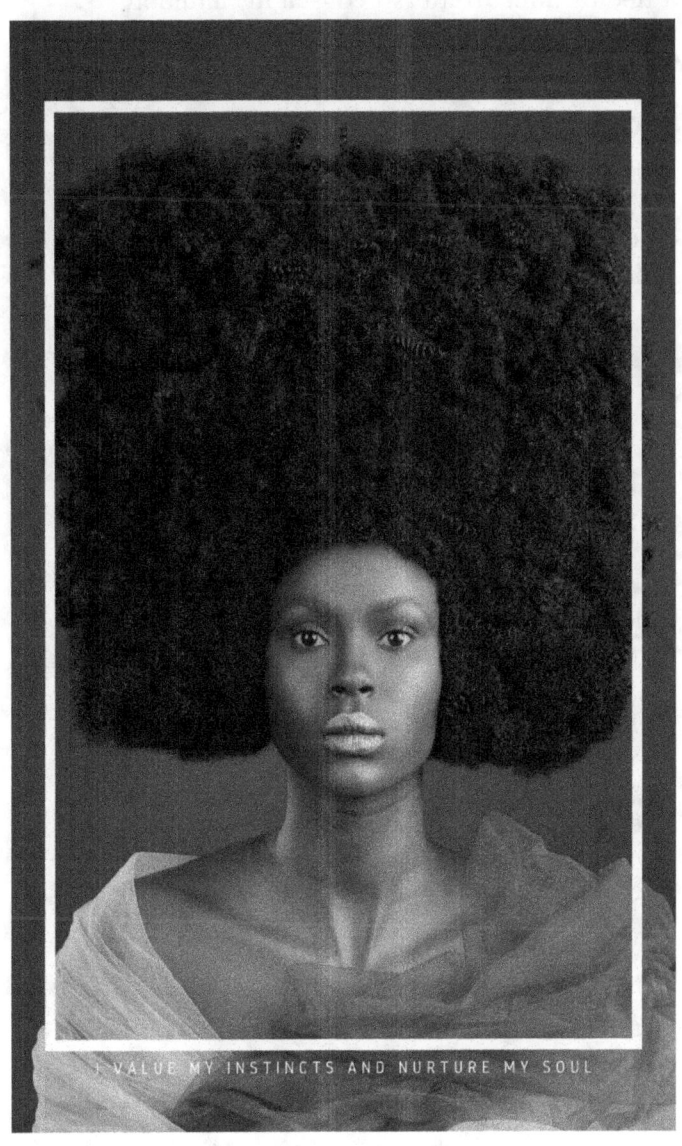

I find the inner truth as I consult my intuition

I express who I am without inhibition

I love myself for me–it's a given, and doesn't have to be earned

I forgive you and you and you… forgiving serves my inner peace.

My inside world reflects into my outside world–I cherish both

My decision is to make my world an amazing place to be alive

My mind is my tool–I use it like a whip to my will

I am a unique person–I am my own me

My strengths are my assets

I express myself thoroughly and honestly

I complete myself without any assistance

I am me, complete and powerful

I have limitless potential

I am my best friend–I am gentle with myself

I remember to dream, confident in my abilities

Fierce, like a panther, I love others passionately

I feel all my feelings, letting even uncomfortable ones through me

I own my self-worth, giving time for rest and relaxation

I enjoy getting better—my journey is perfection

My body gave me my intuition and I listen to it

My beauty expresses itself inside and out

I love my body and everything I do with it

I move fluidly, breezing like an angel through the air, a mermaid in the water, and a goddess in fire

My creative fires are passionate and free

It feels good to be me—I am cared for

My power exists within me, on the inside

I speak and think kindly to myself

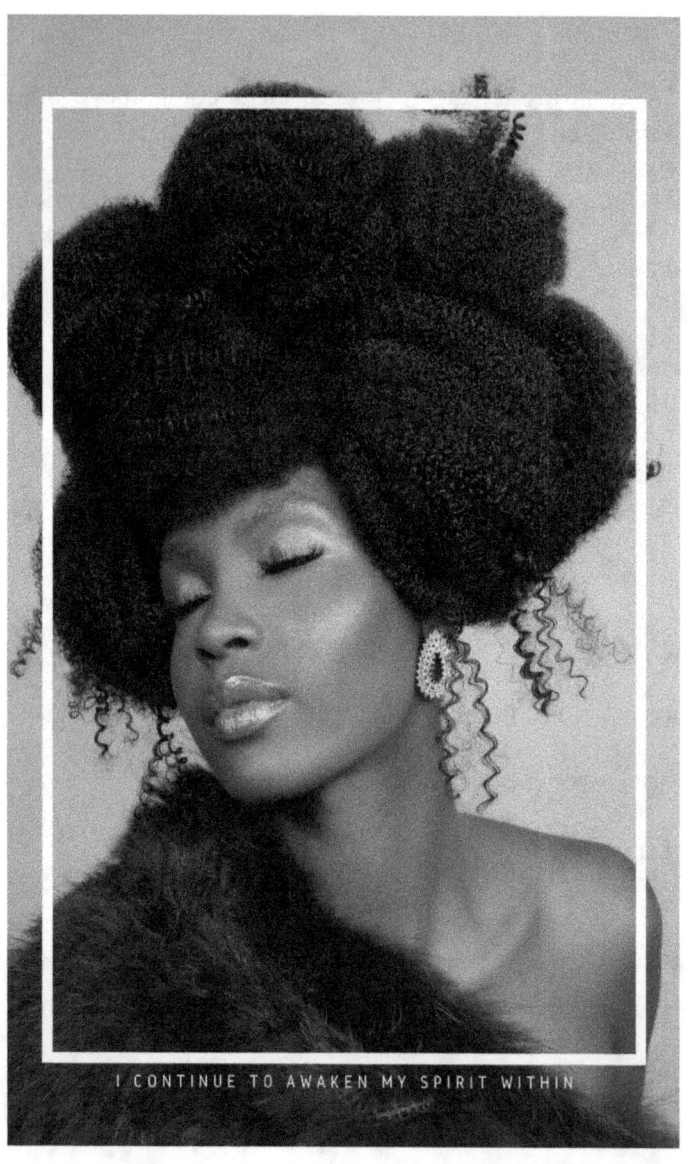
I CONTINUE TO AWAKEN MY SPIRIT WITHIN

What I think of myself is what matters

My completeness includes others–I ask for help and appreciate affections

My feelings inspire me to express my mind and heart

Even when sad, I can handle my feelings

It's ok to feel bad–I love learning from mistakes and owning up to them

My intuition grows and grows as I trust it and use it

When I look in the mirror I see a powerful black queen

My own majesty manifests as I awaken my divine spirit

I love myself endlessly, as my desires are manifested

Who I am is full of abundance and everlasting joy

I provide tenderness for the world and enjoy reaping what I sow

Conclusion

This is the final chapter of the book. We should remember how much work we have done to complete all of these affirmations. If we just read through this for the first time, we should go back, and find ways to *speak* these words. It's worth it to use this book as often as we can–take these words on money, healing, and self-love as a walking bible, the word of a Goddess–she who is worthy of living her dreams.

As a habit, before I leave in the morning, I usually take 5 minutes to myself, and speak into a mirror my daily affirmations. It takes great courage and bravery to face ourselves with expectations of something more. But my dear Goddess, you, the black queen of incredible might and power–we just need to watch ourselves as our lives erupt into fulfilling stories of grandeur and joy. Your destiny is what inspired me to write this, as I found mine in my voice so many years ago.

Life is meant to be lived, fully and completely. Our voice is meant to be heard. Let's respect our words and find integrity in our actions. Let's be mindful as we develop our keen sense of judgment and balance it with our intuitive sense of mercy.

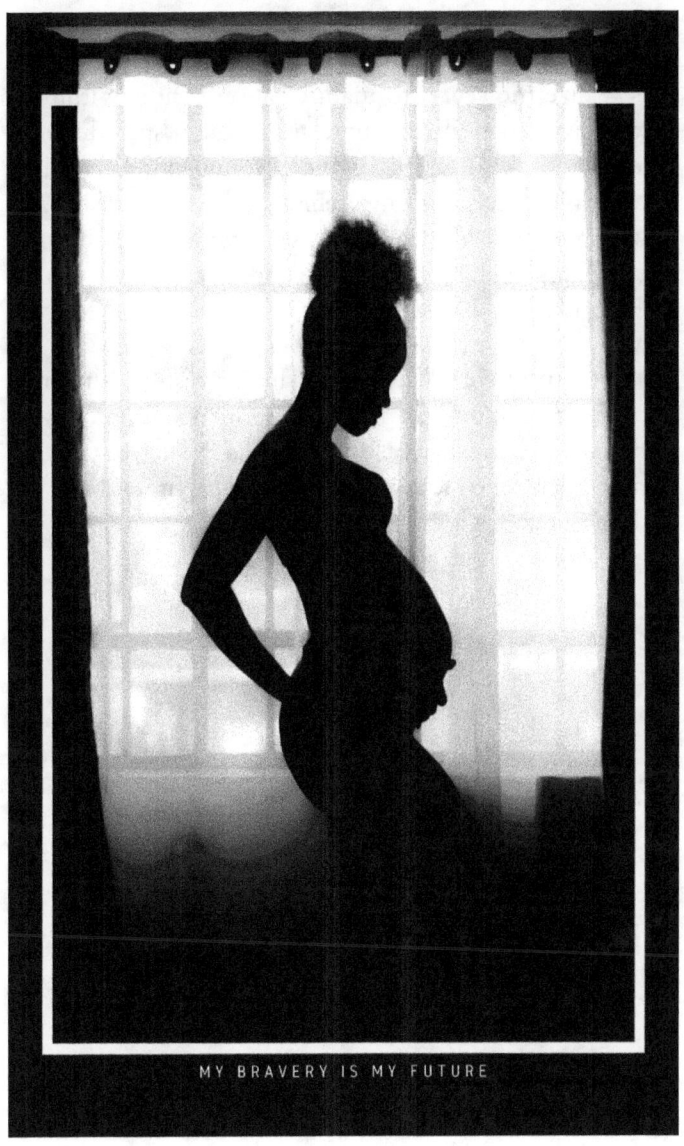

Enjoy collaborating with others and share this book in every way so that we can enlighten them. Most of all, let's realize the secret to manifestation is now within us as we have harmonized ourselves through speaking and listening to these words while forming new thoughts. We should leave nothing behind us as we finish each day. Again, the life we want awaits within–manifesting our dreams to live the life we didn't know we could, starts now.

We at Intuitive Way Publishing would sincerely appreciate your honest review of your experience with these affirmations. Please leave us a 5-star review on Amazon letting us know who you'd recommend this to, with pictures or video.

Powerful Manifestations to Realize the Wisdom of Forgiveness and Your Divine Feminine

Introduction

My pain is not spoken of because they can't hear my cries. The ignorance of my potential reaches beyond what they are capable of seeing. My destiny is truly mine to manifest as I remove the bounds they placed over my mouth so as to speak my heart. What do they know about a successful black woman? Indefinite respect, which I define through my powerful sense of self-respect. This stems from the divine feminine within me and allows me to be my true self.

And so, I have seen the efforts of my mother, and her femininity evokes in me a spiritual warrior. My inner warrior is as fierce as a wolf challenging a bear. The bear is the system, and it is against me, yet I howl and sing, howl and sing. My voice is my divine power because when I speak, my words are felt in homes, on the street, and in the wild. Many historical tales of black women still stir up tears and wet eyes; but do you know the glory of the black woman? My dear, you need not weep anymore for I have found the way to keep my head high, to push on through the limitations that come with being a black woman in this society.

This book of affirmations will delve into the untold pains and unseen tears of black women as we venture on the journey to realize our full potential. You will witness the purities of a black woman in an impure world.

"For the word of God is living and active, sharper than any two-edged sword, piercing to the division of soul and of spirit, of joints and of marrow, and discerning the thoughts and intentions of the heart"

–Hebrews 4:12

With the power of the Word, I will blossom in my elegance and unlock all my chakras. Precious meditation stones and crystals allow me to be fueled by positive energies, radiated forth as my creative energies intertwine within my spirit. Through this energy, I can be understood and heard. Perhaps that is all I yearn for in my lifetime: to be understood, to be heard.

All I want is to discover and fulfill my destiny. I pray that I may plant myself in my rightful place in this world, where I can blossom, and people can witness how powerful I truly am. I learned this from my mother. She and I are witnesses to the assumptions of who I am based on the color of my skin. I do not

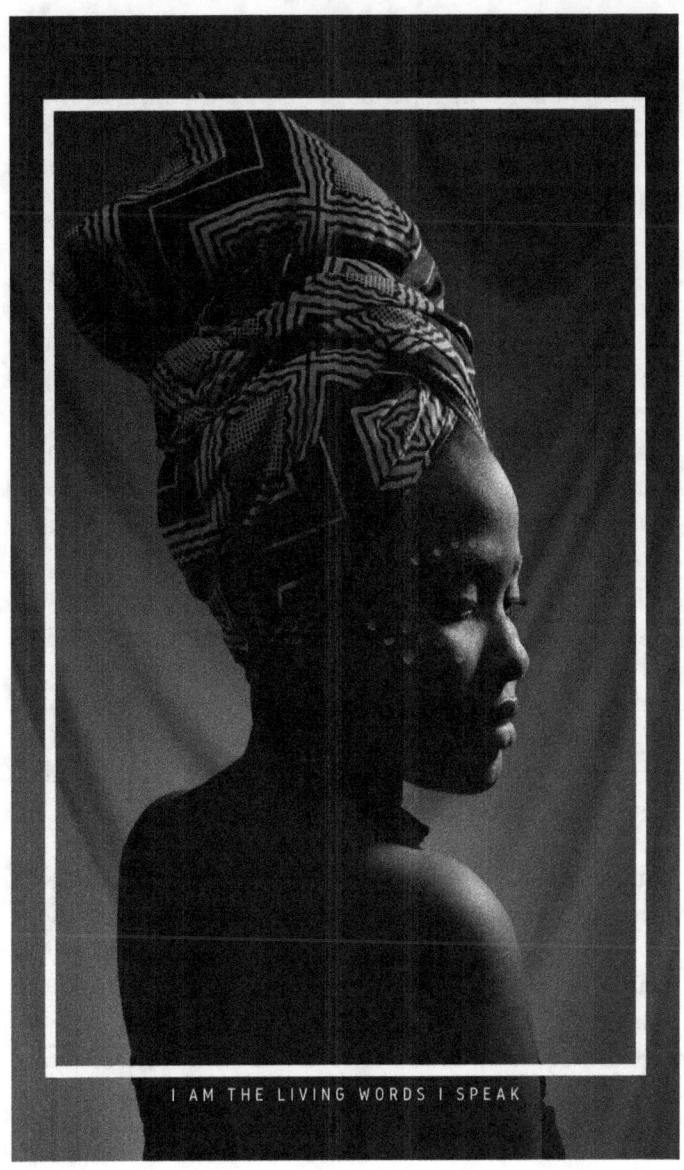

assume I know who I am; instead, I make this journey of self-discovery necessary. I want to reveal my powerful nature with people who take the time to foster it with me. In a world where they attack me for my being, self-love is the greatest defense! I am undefeated as I conquer my destiny.

The best part of my journey is how I have found purpose in embracing my true self through forgiveness. They can judge my scars, but are they aware of the pain the black woman endures? This pain has made me aware of the different energies, both positive and negative, that I am exposed to. Some of the negative energies I have surrounded myself with cannot be changed, and I forgive them with blessings and goodwill. Perhaps when they see me, they already assume who I am and declare my fate; the black woman lives a life of prejudice from the moment she enters this universe. To let prejudice enter my universe is to remember all lessons learned are absorbed through forgiveness. They are so afraid of me, yet they don't know the abundance of love I carry. Yet I still choose to share this love with them.

If they did not fear me, would they still judge me? I know we are meant to accept the flaws of those whom we love. Yes, as a black woman, our flaws are judged. It is as if they have created a false image of what a black woman should look like and how a black woman should behave, and if we do not meet their expectations, then we suffer what they might decide.

Sometimes all it takes is a hug. That single black mother who has to feed the next generation of talent? These black mothers have given birth to some of the most powerful icons to walk among us! Yet, a hug, an embrace, or some kind words—this is all it takes to remind them who nurtured them.

I radiate my mother's divine feminine energy because I inherited it, full of joy. Her ability to survive in a world that only presented her with obstacles casts a ray of light to shine over me. Her feminine energy pulses through her heart and it has taught me to find peace in the world's chaos, through every trial and tribulation. She used her sense of purpose in this world to heal her troubled heart. You know, I am the reason for my mother's efforts. Her warrior spirit exists because of me, and now it is within me. She taught me to endure those who seek to overpower me with words of forgiveness.

Growing up while having to endure the entrenched limitations that this world has for black women has taught us the virtue of our strengths against our weaknesses. We need to pull through the cruelties of injustice with this prayer:

"Do not judge, and you will not be judged. Do not condemn, and you will not be condemned. Forgive, and you will be forgiven."

–Luke 6:37)

Without hypersexualization we can still be powerful. Our divine feminine is the way, as it is beautiful and is an expression of success. It is an expression of who we are in the world, and is met with stares of awe in our graciousness. A black woman's arrival at peace comes through her ability to provide forgiveness to the world's prejudice against her. This inspires the divine feminine, which is the aspect all women share, regardless of whether they are black or not.

This divine feminine is not controversial or unique to one woman. All women are powerful in this way—to conceive, birth, and nurture the next generation. The only door through which humanity may enter for fulfillment regarding intimate love and the fulfillment of breeding is the door of the divine feminine. The door of the woman. This divine right needs to be taught, protected, nourished, and given to be free. This highly potent, natural, God-like

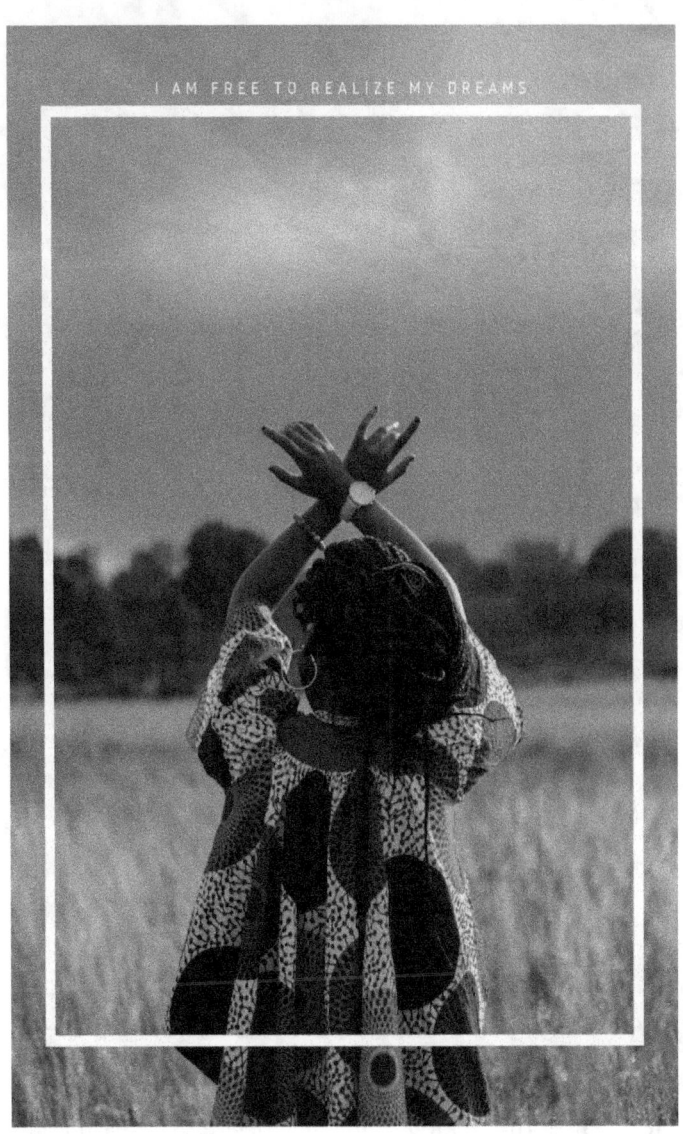

feeling of divinity is to be cherished and respected by women, for women.

Goals

The goals of this book are sevenfold and simple:

1. Find the joy of a black woman in her culture.
2. Shine with beauty in a black woman's skin.
3. Become fully expressive in the way a black woman speaks.
4. Find love for the unique body shape of a black woman.
5. Exude confidence for the intelligence of the black woman.
6. Develop the presence of mind as a successful black woman.
7. Remain committed to healthy lifestyles for the black woman, free from substance abuse.

I, a black woman, am not ashamed of who I am, and I'm enthused at the possibility of my grandiose success. My story can serve as an inspiration to a fellow black woman who may feel as though she does not belong. Her sense of lacking and her desire to belong are because she has yet to meet a person who has seen what she has seen. She searches for a person who has felt what she has felt. This book will comfort her, and its affirmations will help her to realize that being a black woman is a special gift. She will know how her divine feminine is far greater than the power of the wicked who tell us that being a black woman isn't enough. Weep not, my dear black women, for these affirmations bring us solace.

Chapter 4:

Affirmations to Accept Peace and Stand Powerful

I have to find my inner peace so that I am able to be at peace with others. Even though they have wronged me through their naive and manipulated minds, I need to find equilibrium for my emotions so that I do not lose touch with my mercy and grace. I am more than the scars that remind others of my past. My present is filled with abundance, joy, and love, and I share this energy with those who have judged me for being a black woman, because this act is evidence that we are able to coexist with one other.

I hope there comes a day where they don't just remember me for being a black woman, but also that they see me as an ordinary human being, just like the rest of us; they should see that I also bleed red, have a soul, and enjoy ambition. I too might be just another black woman, but with these affirmations I redefine the black woman. Just watch as they see me differently, seeing as I have forgiven them before

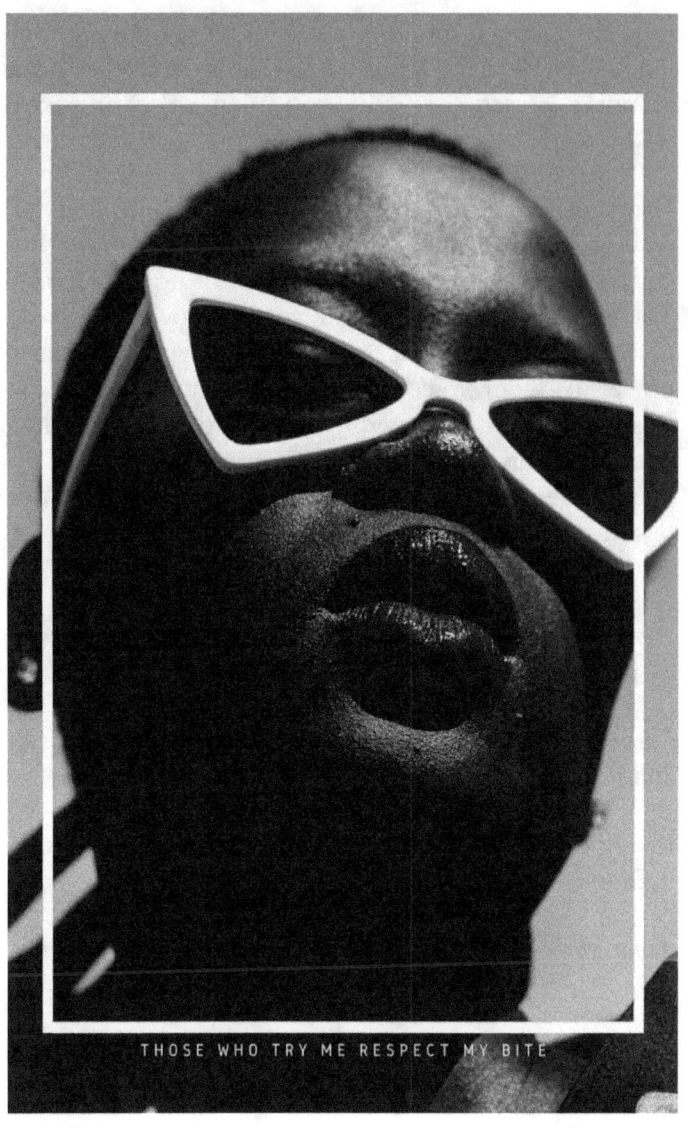

they have judged me. A world without prejudice is one where we live together to be appreciative of our feminine presence regardless of skin color or sexual orientation.

For those listening, follow the prompts. If you are reading, remember to repeat this not just mentally, but with your voice. You can make this profound change! The world is waiting, and you have the power! Use your voice and believe in what makes you ultimately powerful—your voice and your projections of fire! Do this in front of the mirror, as you drive, while riding your bike, through mountainous terrain, as you put on your makeup, or in the shower. I believe in you. Your destiny is yours and yours only. Find it within yourself, use your words, and repeat these now

I coexist faithfully, observing my mystery may not yet be understood

I forgive those who prejudge me based on stereotypes and pop culture.

Prejudices may attempt to trigger me, but they don't define who I am

Their prejudice can be changed if they can experience me

I reveal to myself my own powerful ability as I recognize others affirming theirs

I forgive to inspire people to understand black women

I am worthy of being heard. My story is unique, and my perspective is divine to me.

I love sharing who I am with others because I learn more about myself through others

Forgiveness is an opportunity to build faith in humanity

I love the black queen I'm becoming, and I want to share this radiance with others

I share my blessings to help others appreciate their own blessings

They are free to think as they wish, and I, the black woman, am wise to forgive with abundance and good will

I overcome judgment with faith in my inner chambers—the chambers of my heart—where I am in control

There are doors that will eventually open for me

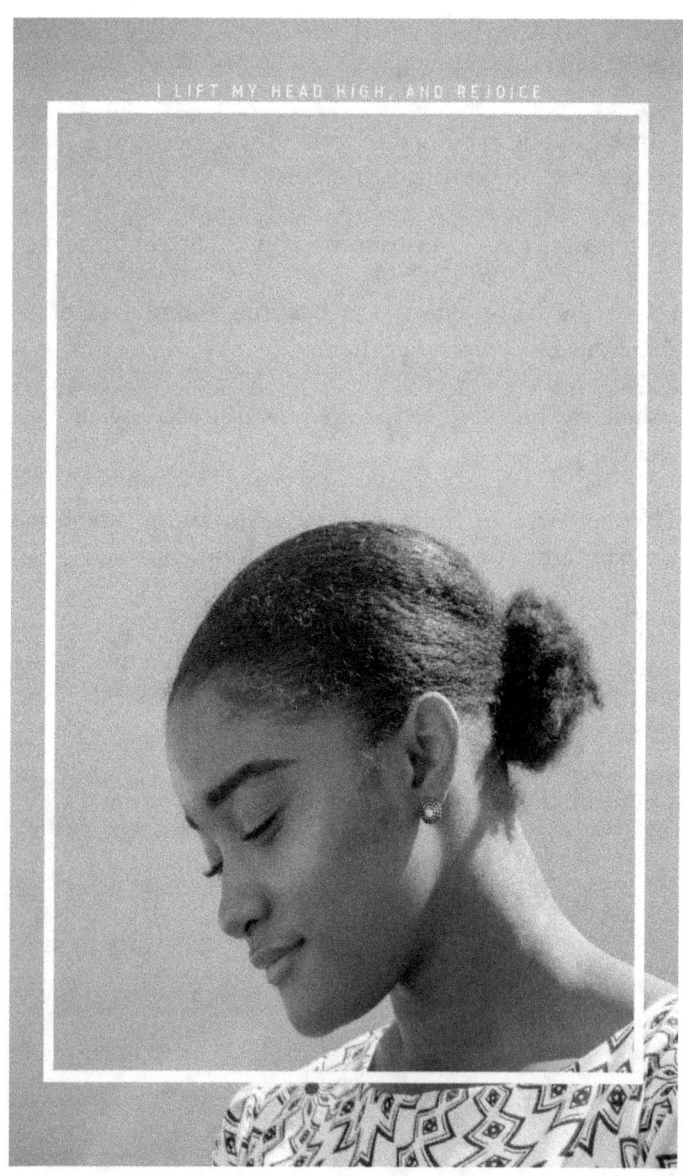

I position myself to reach my destiny, and it's my responsibility to take action with the life I'm given

My survival is my decision, just like anyone's is. I choose a path that values my desires, dreams, and goals

I take action to inspire righteousness in the face of injustice, goodwill in the face of ignorance, and empathy in the face of shame

The trauma they left us with is nothing! I am powerful to heal and unafraid to succeed

Their judgment of my skin color is their inability to acknowledge the beauty before their eyes

Black is beautiful, and I bathe in the water that makes my essence glow

I see no flaw with my skin color because the cracks within the skin have been mended together by my gracious aura

Black is noticeable because it's unique in its own color and fashion

Black is full of history, heritage, and culture

I stand as tall as a tree with deep roots, with pride for who I am

I inspire other black women by owning up to my responsibility within my culture, my language, and my fashion

The diary of a black woman is filled with emotion that can be depicted through art

Our artistic way of expressing ourselves brings about a peace in our demeanor

The music I listen to makes me dance the night away in amazement of how special I am

I am composed of eternal greatness, and I will embrace my victory, for I have suffered many losses

Black history is filled with black women who died standing firm in what they believe in, which spurs hope inside me

My beliefs give me self-worth, and my code of conduct seeks to find mutual respect with others

I am an element of peace, and I seek to integrate as a whole to unite with other peaceful black women

My standing tall and proud motivates other black women to find similar power within themselves

I am able to inspire others and help guide them toward their greater purpose

I band together with other black women—together we find peace and build strength

I share my voice with other black women, and it is powerful—we are impassioned to forgive

I accept me for the black woman I am, and I appreciate others who offer affection to my cause

I accept my true nature, and I feel happily independent

The true nature of the black woman is mighty, glorious, and worthy of worship

Every black woman has a calling to her divine feminine nature, and every black woman can achieve it, regardless of prejudice

I am here to lead and walk among them as we all journey toward our greater purpose

I sharpen my wit and will to thrive with the help of my black sisters

I feel empathy for my sister, as she must rise through the stereotypical shame cast on her as a black woman

I want all black women to find their power and use it to determine their rightful place in this world

I am free to live my life to the fullest

Even when my surroundings are in turmoil, my peace will not be shaken

I choose to have serenity in my everyday life

I release all that worries me and seek refuge in my feminine graces

I let the opinions of others wash over me without concern

I have the freedom to embrace my power

I am intact with my inner peace

I attract harmony into my life

My power comes from within

Everything I need is already within me

I radiate glorious feminine energy

I always support my fellow black sisters

I go with my own flow, even if the world wants me to swim the other way

I welcome judgments without fear because I have already forgiven them

I am a positive influence to the world around me

I let any hate and negativity pass by—I take no offense as a black woman

My existence as a black woman serves me—it is my life to enjoy

I am led by, and I lead with love. Just love

I freely speak my truth and live in it

I will rise no matter how many times I fall

I create a safe space within me, where I am wholly receptive to myself and my femininity

I welcome opportunity and strive to take advantage of it

My creative power lets me create a better life for myself

I can overcome anything

I have everything I need to become successful

I stand strong in my power

Shame is my sword of empathy—I understand the color of my skin is its sharp edge

My thoughts are positive, my soul nourished, my body cared for

I define me as a powerful black woman, regardless of circumstances

My hair is curly, and its texture is coarse—these are my beautiful features

I am kind to myself, and I notice the kindness in others

I process love, so I appreciate the finer things in life like tenderness and romance

I am confident about my feminine side, and I rejoice in being a woman

I determine my own destiny, and I work to manifest it

All I have to do is be myself

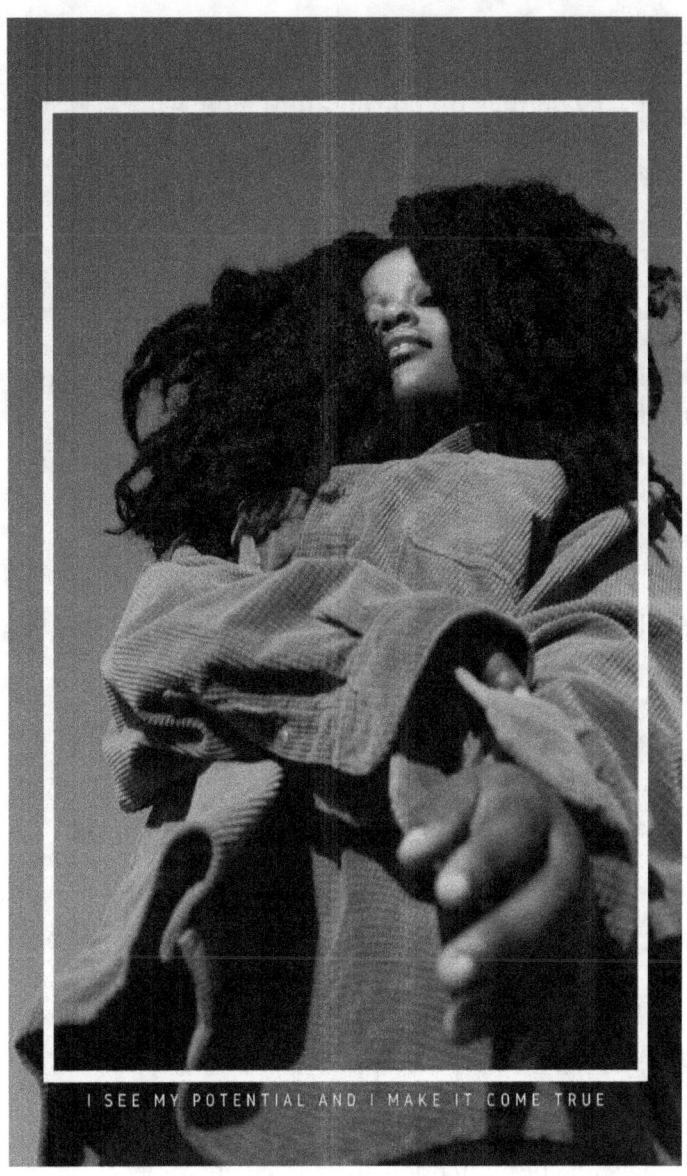

I do not have to change who I am for the world

I speak faithfully from my heart to those who will listen

I accept the love I think I deserve, and I deserve divine love from the heavens above

I celebrate my culture and heritage, taking pride in my role as a black woman

I am divinely blessed by my mother and her mother before her

Abundance is my birthright

I am valuable to myself, powerful as I remain present

I speak up and take action when I am unjustly served. I respect myself

I am capable of manufacturing my own happiness

I empathize with others, and through these relationships, I am healthy

I release all fear as I seize my power

I am ambitious and set my goals—powerful are my intentions

My feminine nature is peaceful, capable of balancing creation and destruction

I have the best intentions for myself and others

I speak to my fellow black women, and I preach that they stay powerful, stay true, and stay beautiful

Chapter 5:

Affirmations to Embrace Self-Love and to Find Justice in Forgiveness

The Angelite stone not only helps me find peace and protects me, but it enhances the energy of self-love within me. Angelite is a soft lilac-blue stone meant to relieve tension and calm anger. It's a very spiritual stone, allowing us to connect to celestial bodies to request healing to take place. Angelite can also be paired with Kunzite to ensure self-love.

When it comes to justice, we should practice forgiveness as a means of achieving justice. Thus, it is better to forgive than to seek revenge. Thanks to the public safety measures and stones like Angelite, black women can still feel protected.

I love myself and I know that I am destined to be more than just the face of a divine mother. I see no issue with the color of my skin, and I search for every opportunity to express who I am as a person. My self-expression is not an attack on society. Instead, it is my way of announcing my presence in this world. I announce who I am, and I listen to others who do the same; for it is with equality that we recognize the excellence of the world. Am I wrong for expecting my forgiveness to be rewarded with a round of applause? I deserve my respect as a black woman, and I will influence others to be great as well.

I am beautiful and wonderfully made

Others who seek comfort in me will find it—my ability to forgive is endless and limitless

I look in the mirror and marvel at how amazing I am

I forgive to inspire people to understand black women

The world will experience me at my fullest expression—I prepare the world and I prepare myself for this coming moment

I won't dwell on my pain and heartache anymore. Through wisdom I find strength; through forgiveness I find courage

Prejudice denies them from seeing our true majesty—but it's okay because I forgive them

Forgiveness is a long road because I measure it in doses. I don't want to forget my boundaries

Baseless opinions of me breeze over my cheeks and cool my hot black skin

I inspire greatness in all who are ready to experience it—I have the energy for it

I am noticed and I am found—I face the challenges of black women and I tackle the norms

I am able to forgive, and I do—I feel healed through forgiveness

I am recognized because I am worthy—my greatness is the throne of my intuition

My comfort in my intuitive graces allows me to forgive those for being fearful

Fierce is my love for myself, as I have dominion of my feminine powers, ready to influence the next generation

My leadership is my path, narrow as it may be. It goes unrecognized by many who aren't ready to forgive themselves

I do not judge wrongdoings haphazardly; I am willing to show forgiveness

The leadership of the black woman is divine and perfect, staying true to a life of purpose

I have divine power within me to do miraculous things

I am a bundle of wonder and joy, so unique and original that I recognize how legends are made

Place me in a high position—I am responsible for being fair and wise

Cowardice, hypocrisy, and prejudice confront me, but I have powerful wisdom, charms of forgiveness, and feminine sweetness

Faith makes black women tough, but with the wisdom of forgiveness, I am prepared to get tougher

The black woman I am is precisely immaculate

The immaculate powers of creation rest within the beautiful feminine divinity within me—there is nothing to stress about

I try to help all women, making my mark with my beautiful black skin inspiring a divine toughness

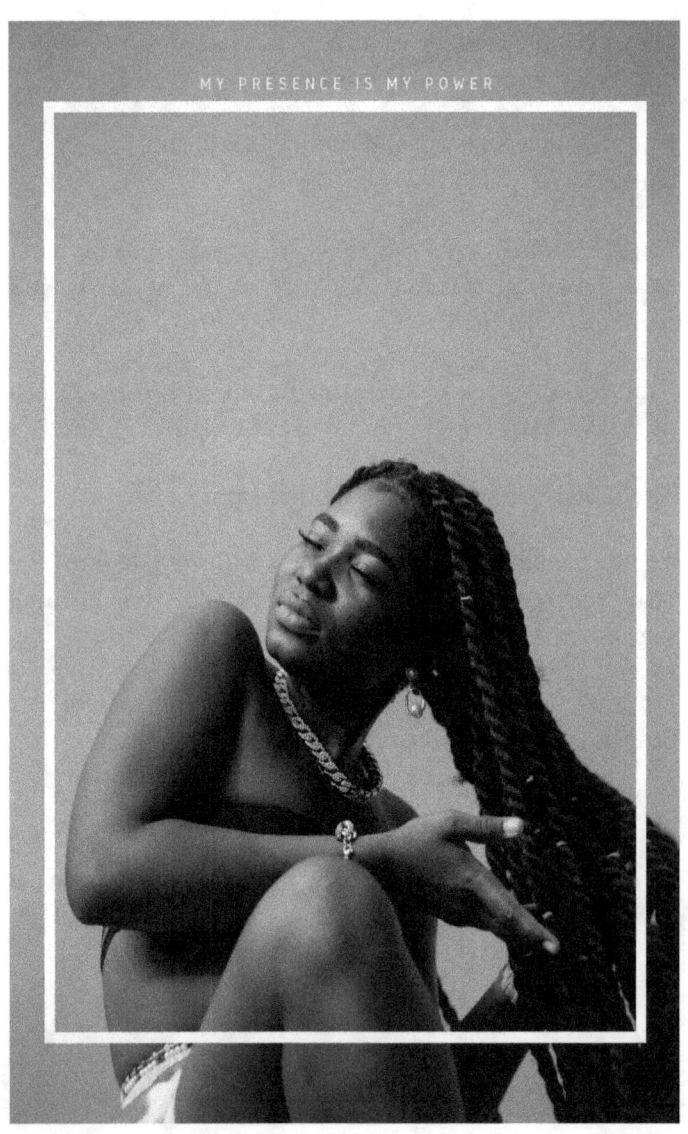

Just because I am not favored by the crowds doesn't mean I'm not favored by my divinity

I love my body and I kiss it every day in appreciation

My body is my life's work of art—I have unlimited potential to work on it

I recognize the ultimate love of God is within my divine feminine body, but no one is entitled to this sacred body except whom I choose

I treat my black body with love and care and inspire others to do the same with theirs

I am a black woman with cosmic, divine intelligence—swimming in heavenly thoughts, I beckon the good will of others

I use any knowledge of self-love to forgive, using humility and a pure heart

I rise above expectations without question—my bravery heals me

I have dreams of being successful, of earning achievements in my name—self-love is no gamble. I seek not fortune or fame

The clarity of my inner faith defines me, setting a foundation for a life of magnificence

I adorn myself with elegance

I am not dependent on a man for money. I am independent and I can make my own money

My identity as a black woman is set by my self-image—I have the power to redefine and refine myself every day to get better and better at being me

Being great and achieving greatness is my destiny to manifest

Confidence is the aura I embody with every step forward I take, and it helps me let go of the past without fear of mistakes

I listen and hear those who are arrogant and gloat—my ability to forgive lets my inner peace remain undisturbed

I can be good to those who've wronged me because I am capable of forgiving

The merits of my forgiveness are not measured by those who accept it, but by my ability to give it

Being a black woman requires patience and wisdom—tolerating the lesser of two evils requires generous faith in forgiveness

When others weep on my shoulders, I hear their pain and respect their plight—I accept my role in the journey of acquiring wisdom in life

My voice, my culture, and my name carry my black skin when others are blind, enlightening them to respect my feminine powers

As I forgive others, I truly forgive myself too—justice is love served with divine wisdom

I define my future every day as I speak my purpose, and let my amazing feminine powers purify my intentions

I live to love and I love to love because some people need my love

We all need love, and sometimes the best source of love is ourselves

Every person struggles. By aligning our energies with our life's purpose, we rise together above any prejudice that divides us

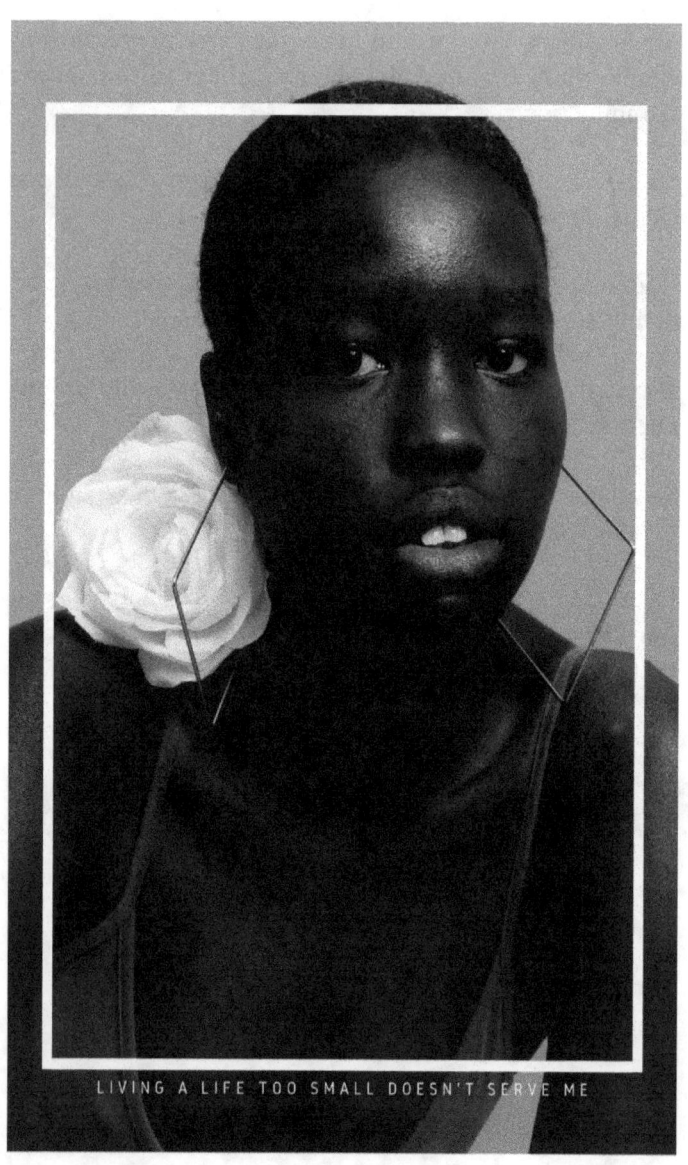

When we are born to be conceived as enemies, we have not forgiven ourselves. When we forgive ourselves, our friends will be found everywhere

In the end, my divine feminine is my grace, and the good I do with it is what passes on

Being unique is me acknowledging my innocence—being unique is me deciding to be someone

My forgiving heart beats for me and for my time on Earth. My life as a black woman is a story of divine blessings

Who has felt the rays of the sun? I have, the black woman I am. I am enough to enjoy it

Being myself is humility in action—it's the best thing I can do

Being myself is kindness in action—I treat others the way I want to be treated

My hair and my dreads magnify the importance of my beautiful, divine wisdom through my black body

My lips and my hips show voluptuousness that enhance my sexual presence through my black body

My eyes are my prize, and my delicate thighs communicate my power and majesty through my black body

My words and my slang teach me to remember my thang as I handle the sounds and vibrations through my black body

I accept the blessings of my sisters, and desire to be authentic to them too

I deserve to let my light shine—living a small life of mediocrity may comfort others but let them be forgiven as I leave my comfort zone

I determine my self-worth, not others

I am proud of my achievements and celebrate them with others who respect me

I have always had my feminine powers within me—realizing my potential to use them is my life's work

A black woman who thinks positively is equal to any woman. Knowing so is both powerful and wise

A black woman who sees the good in herself has begun to mirror the allure of her feminine mystery on others

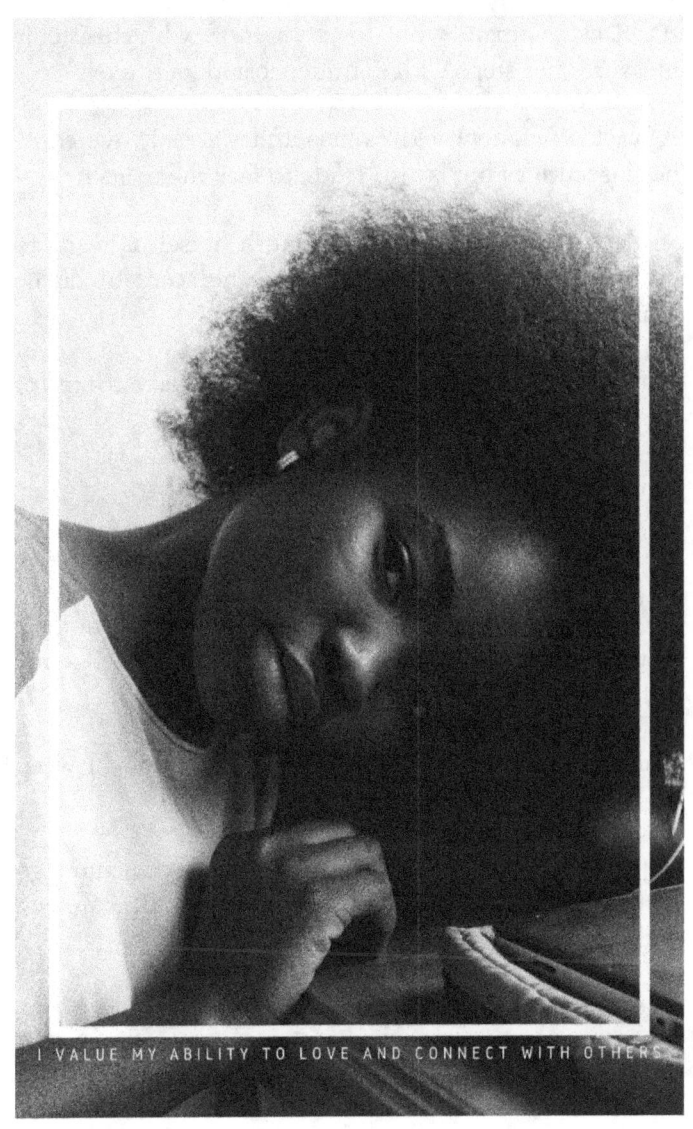

A black woman who loves herself wholeheartedly measures her steps with confidence and gratitude

A black woman who loves herself has already overcome her insecurities but is also ready to face them again

A black woman who is confident in herself is ready to be as alluring as perfume, leaving the scent of divine inhalation as a mark of divine fulfillment

Doubt is released from within me and I make room for positive beliefs

Even on bad days I nurture myself

I adore my melanated skin

To seek validation is to choke on confidence not yet found. I welcome the journey to fully acknowledge my potential

I forgive myself over my emotional hang-ups—I weep no longer and breathe easier

I appreciate those who love me for who I am, and I go further to love me for who I am capable of being, yes, with the love of others too

The deeper I go inside the chambers in my heart, the more powerful is the mystery of my femininity

Chapter 6:

Affirmations to Unearth the Divine Feminine Within Me, Because We Know We Are Powerful Black Women

Three chosen stones—Kunzite, Clear Quartz, and Angelite—work together to process forgiveness in my divine feminine aspects. I am a nurturer, and I am filled with feminine powers. I am able to use my energy to help groom others as they nurture their feminine aspects too. When I nurture, I raise up spirits, and set passions ablaze. My perspective is to build bonds of trust that root down into the individual, where she may become independent, free of my influence. As we nurture, we hope to develop people into those ready to be righteous amid chaos, and not to expose the world to pain. My divine feminine reminds me of the healing powers I

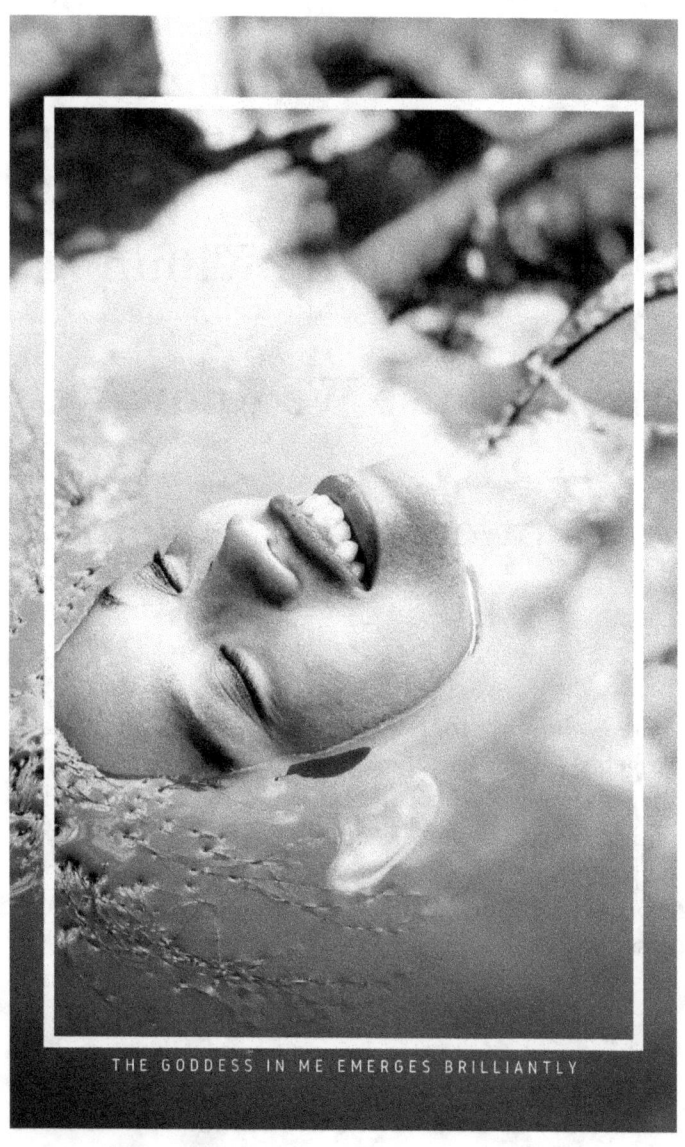

possess. It reminds me that my voice is enough. Everything divine in my holy womb reminds me of the healing powers I possess. It reminds me that my voice is enough. When I speak my words, I enshrine happiness as an outcome of my intentions.

My voice is no more a weapon than these high-frequency stones, each a million years old. I choose to uplift those who can't fight the fatigue of conceiving for such a long period of time. My actions guide anyone to follow suit, so if I am being honest, I guide them and receive the same honesty in return. I lend my ear to listen to those who are misguided and offer what I know to be true to give them value and structure. I say no more than what I know to be true. When I have nothing good to say, I know it is better to say nothing. That's why my divine feminine, my cosmic womb, teaches me to be compassionate. The black woman is tempted to be undermined by dismay, pettiness, and bigotry, but when her heart is filled with compassion, she busts down those walls of ill intentions.

In my community I seek peace where all might be powerful. This corner of faith is built on togetherness and laughter, lightheartedness, and dreams—so much happiness that we enjoy getting a little busy.

"Strength and dignity are her clothing, and she laughs at the time to come. She opens her mouth with wisdom, and the teaching of kindness is on her tongue"

—Proverbs 31:25-26

I am capable of nurturing others by sharing my views, experiences, and knowledge

I seek to teach what I've learned because it helps me learn that I know what I know, and that when someone reaches in faith for help, I am ready to help them

I am powerful enough to reach my objectives according to my desires

The energy I possess of my divine feminine is holy and sacred, but also sensual and fun

Sacred energy resides within me, and I nourish it with playfulness

Black as I am, I am aligned with all things divinely feminine that feed my soul

I release all that no longer serves me to my highest good

I am in control of my life and can choose what is best for me

My body is sacred and I highly value it

I am grateful for my body and its sensual parts that allow me to fully enjoy my human experience

I creatively express my femininity

I am divinely guided and protected

I can do anything I set my mind to, regardless of circumstances

I have the ability to bring about a positive change to the world around me

Abundance is attracted to me; I am a magnetic black woman

I am a powerful, sensual, and divine black woman

My sexuality is embraced with open arms, and it is not something to be ashamed of

I attentively listen to my intuition

I was born from greatness, and I will carry this greatness with me throughout my days

I am attuned with my inner magic

I am the universe in human form

I am a living, breathing goddess

I can be brave and gentle at the same time

I am aligned with my highest good

I honor the frequent cycles that my body goes through

My black beauty is divine and ethereal

I love freely and with an open heart

I am open to receiving and giving pleasure

I am the living royalty that is preached of in the Bible

I deserve nothing but the best of the best

I am admired by others for the divine will in me to manifest my destiny

Cosmic energy flows through my veins

I manifest my destiny with intuitive efforts

My energy is my life—my life is valuable

Kindness radiates in my presence

Vigilant in my heart, I trust my intuition to know I am safe and secure with others around me

My energy radiates like the sun, warming the stones under my feet

I have a daily habit of going one level deeper inside as I seek fulfillment in my feminine prowess

I relate to the conqueror who seeks intimate self-expression

My creativity is fruitful with endless elaborations. I create and innovate with ease

I enjoy the miracles of life, the novelty of experience, and the presence of a caring heart

I touch and embrace to communicate with others in ways that words cannot

All that I desire is intimate to me, and I only share what I want with those I trust

What I lack in experience I make up for in bravery

I set my goals now so that when I look back after five years, I will be happy that I did

In five years, these affirmations will still be just as powerful, only many layers deeper in understanding

I proceed faithfully in my life, knowing that I deserve to earn my keep and my independence

I am powerful. I protect both myself and others with the shelter I keep, which is my home

I am powerful. I treat myself well, decorating and loving my home. It nurtures me and all who are invited to enter

I am powerful. I color my life to accentuate my style, my black body, my culture, and my heritage

I welcome my feminine habits to nurture and love my black skin, my black face, my black body, and my black style

I am realizing the masterpiece of black women everywhere—the mystery of our divine femininity

Any man who seeks to partner with me needs to realize my feminine prowess

I don't wait for perfect moments. I create them

I don't complain. I originate circumstances

When things get difficult, I go a layer deeper

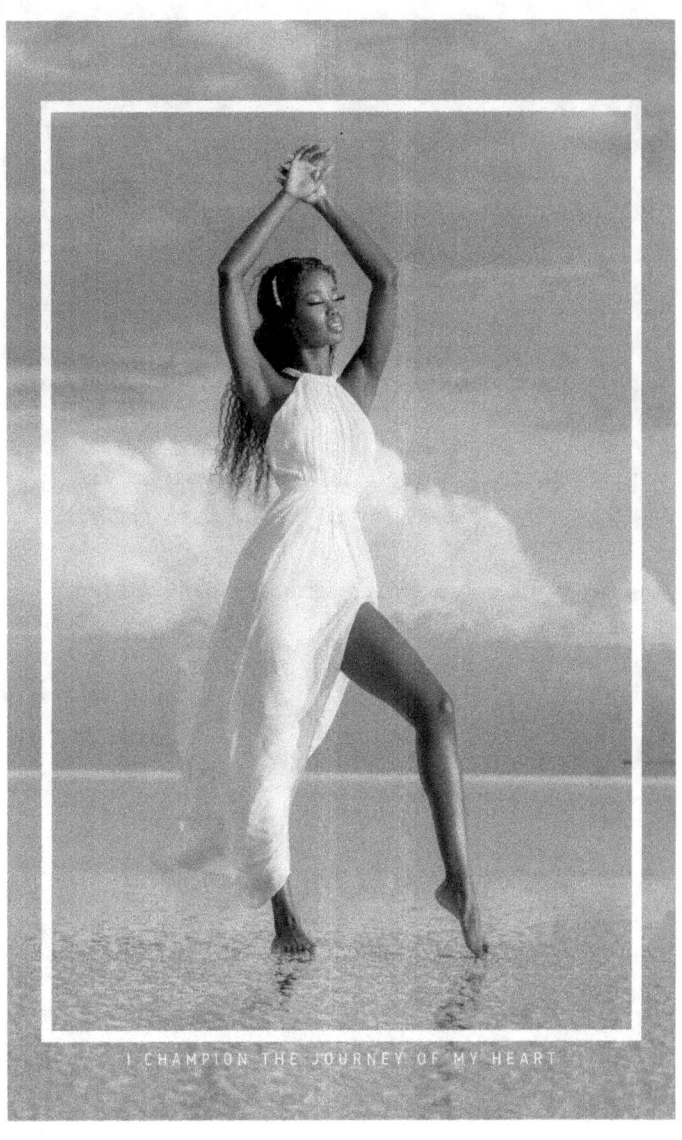

When I forgive myself and others for our difficulties, I remember to celebrate our triumphs

Right now, the black woman is triumphant

Right now, the black woman is rich in serenity and love

Right now, my divine feminine energy spills over and uplifts others

Right now, the black woman is born more beautiful than ever before

A black woman needs to rest only after her heart is satisfied

A satisfied black woman is settled in her own feminine divinity

Conclusion

The long and gruesome history of black women remains a heartbreaking tale. But despite these misfortunes of prejudice, we are passing the tests of time and learning to triumph as a tribe. With everything that the world has thrown at us, we have chosen to be resilient, and we keep our heads held high as we realize the true power within the divinity of every black woman, especially when it comes to taking on the responsibility of seeking out the life we want to live. Our ability to forgive starts as we forgive ourselves—it's okay to want what we want. Black women are blessed to have beautiful black skin, the divine touch, and Afro-textured hair, so we should nourish what makes us us every day.

These affirmations, along with my own story and that of my sisters, will help unite and uplift black women all over the world. Through this we are learning to manifest a new reality—one in which we are realizing just how magical the black woman is.

Together we can make the world realize just how magical the black woman is.

> *"I praise you, for I am fearfully and wonderfully made.*
> *Wonderful are your works; my soul knows it very well"*
>
> *—Psalm 139:14*

Remember Your Inner Child, Perfect Your Self-Image, and Ignite the Fire of Sex

Introduction

Affirmations are statements that release us from the shackles of unwanted thoughts and feelings. They have the power to give us the extra push to keep going when we feel like giving up. The power that words of affirmation have on us is monumental. Affirmations teach us how to talk, how to think, and how to find better feelings for ourselves. A lot of affirmations that we find in this book will be statements that are completely new to us. However, this does not mean that we should hesitate to speak to them. Oh no! You see, affirmations work as a blueprint, letting us know exactly how we need to think and feel about ourselves. When we begin to know this (oh my!), we will then be able to attract the same to us. With such encouraging behavior inside our hearts and minds, these affirmations will become the truth for us.

These affirmations work in many spheres of our life. In this book, we cover affirmations to remember our inner child, perfect our self-image, and ignite the fire of sex. We are all welcome to use these affirmations in any way we please, but in this order, we emerge from the past into a healing space of peace, develop

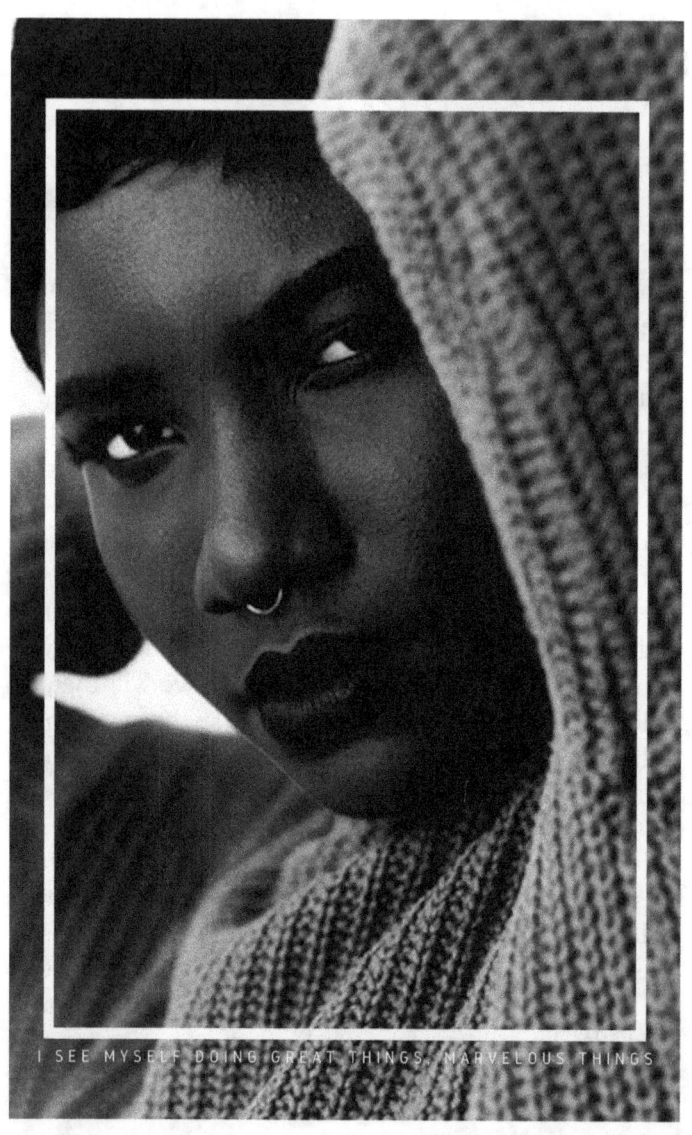

I SEE MYSELF DOING GREAT THINGS, MARVELOUS THINGS

a vision for ourselves to plan for the future, and enjoy the present moment for all its worth. I recommend you speak them out loud in the home, in the car, or meditate on them as mantras in your mind or your journal before you face your day. This way, whenever we are found up against any challenges, we can refresh our memory on the mindset from these affirmations. As black women, as sisters, we need to stick together to enlighten each other on the things we learn in this journey. Affirmations played a vital role in helping my ambitions take root and flourish. So, I would love to see my fellow black women come to realize their fullest potential through these helpful words.

There is great power in the manner in which we identify as a woman. As black women, a lot of ideas in the world exist to bring us down. Unless we find the innocent novelty of our inner child and combine it with the sharp wit of our self-knowledge, we may begin believing the lies that society uses to belittle us. We need to re-channel ourselves towards what we want to believe and achieve in this one life of ours. After all, when we believe in ourselves, we have the creative juices flowing inside of us, and it doesn't matter what others think. Take this precious moment to commit to unlocking the loving fire of passion with affirmations that I present in this book. You will not only find your ability to heal from past traumas but also speak from a wonderful place of splendor and joy as if you are using the creative verb for the first time like children do. You will resolve issues you didn't know you had and see a future for yourself with happiness and harmony in abundance. You will learn the vital importance of self-awareness and acceptance—releasing judgment of any personal flaws. Of course, any invitations to the bedroom will be well beyond the subject of taboo and deep into satisfaction, including the fulfillment of intimate desire and the practice of heavenly adorations of ecstasy. Oh yes, it's great to be a black woman.

Chapter 7:

Affirmations to Remember Your Inner Child

> *Children are a heritage from the Lord,*
> *offspring a reward from him.*
>
> *—Psalm 127:3*

Let's think, breathe, move and remember the little girl we used to be. Her thoughts, her dreams, her aspirations! Perhaps she had no care in the world, nothing but hope and joy for the future. This innocence can sometimes come flooding back, reminding us how precious the present moment is. As black women, we rarely stop to think and assess how great we are for having made it to this point in our lives without being brainwashed by prejudice. Our childhood is what prepared us, and the memory of our inner child will continue to enrich us as we nurture each other towards the future. A woman who is strongly in line with her inner child is a powerful being. This doesn't mean we shouldn't grow up, hardly so! We simply must preserve this

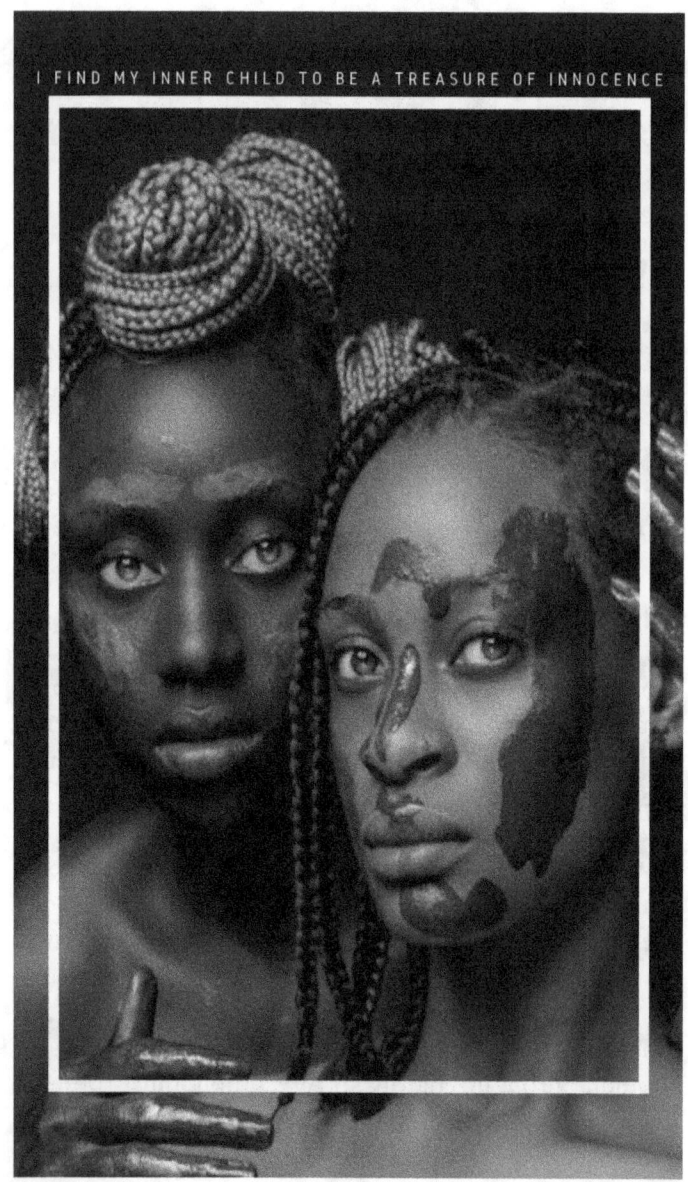

I FIND MY INNER CHILD TO BE A TREASURE OF INNOCENCE

childlike attitude and remark on its novelty. Let's do so with these affirmations.

So, what could reconnection with our inner child bring us now in adulthood?

- self-awareness
- healing
- empowerment
- change

It does not matter our age—it is not too late to get in touch with our inner child. It will bring us relief through self-awareness. We will be able to discern what is right, and what isn't right for each of us. Once we understand any traumas which came from the vulnerable stages of our childhood, we can abide in healing energy to leave those pains behind. We will also be empowered to re-spark the curiosity that our inner child used to have for life. We will also be able to identify pattern behaviors that need to change as we embark on transforming our lives.

For those listening, follow the prompts. If you are reading, remember to repeat this not just mentally, but with your voice. You can do it, girl; this is a profound change! The world is waiting, and you have the power! Use your voice and believe in what makes you ultimately powerful–your voice and your projections of fire!

I am in touch with the needs of my inner child.

Through my child-like presence, I make positive memories

I possess many talents, and I nurture them all with love.

I comfort my inner child and work through fears.

Together with my inner child, my life is renewed, refreshed, invigorated.

I am loved as I am.

I am loved for who I truly am.

I can take constructive criticism.

I can make mistakes; they help me grow.

I am able to approach any challenge in my way.

I am a clever black woman.

I listen to my heart and speak boldly – I've learned to know myself.

Mistakes are lessons learned – I get better from them.

I can do anything I set my mind on.

I am a loving friend.

I am kind.

I allow negative emotions to come and go – I breathe through them.

Where others fail me, I can meet my own needs.

I am willing to grow.

The spirit of my inner child shines through my personality.

I'm pleased with myself.

My feelings and thoughts are significant.

I am sufficient.

I am capable of being authoritative without being aggressive.

I'm one-of-a-kind and extraordinary.

I know what is correct and what is incorrect.

I am capable of standing up for what I believe in.

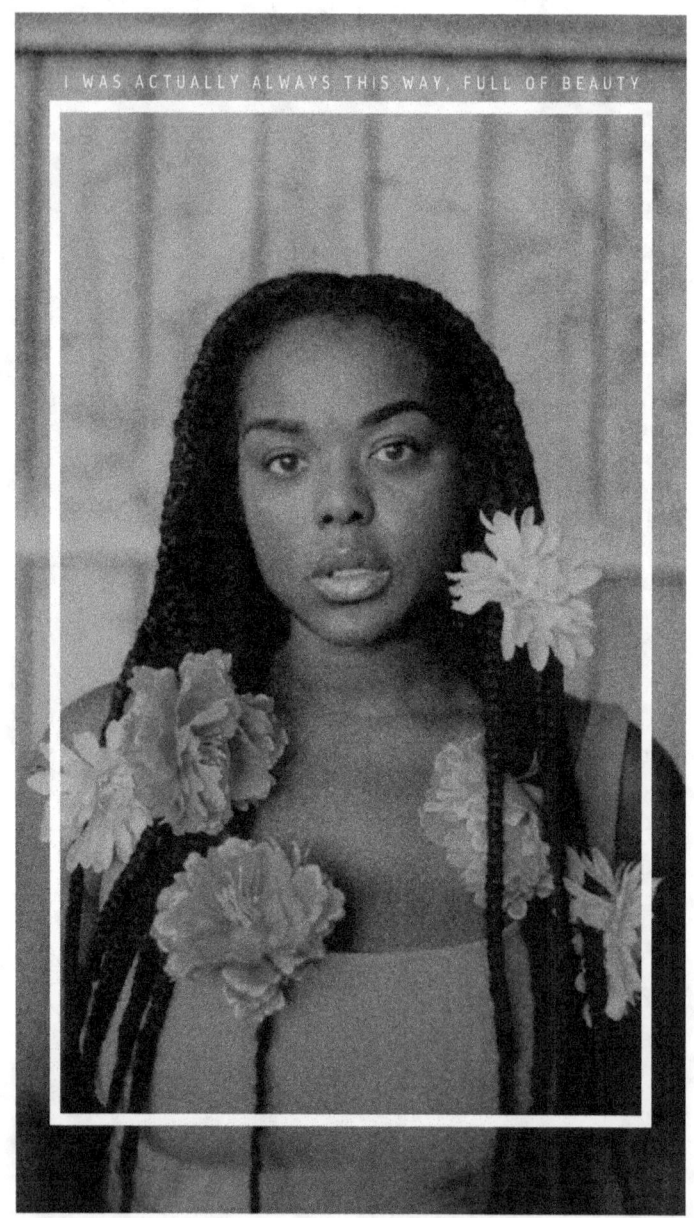

It is my character, not my beauty, that is important.

I am capable of speaking out when someone is mistreating another individual.

I am capable of working hard to reach my objectives.

I am capable of learning everything I set my mind to.

I have the ability to affect positive change in the world.

It is OK to take a break.

I've got a lot to offer.

My body is mine, and I have the ability to define its bounds.

It is OK to seek assistance.

I can perform tiny acts of kindness to help others.

I am not weak because I seek guidance.

I'm an artist.

It's okay for me to experience all of my emotions.

I adore myself as much as I adore others.

Our differences make us unique.

I have the ability to turn a negative situation around.

When I've done something I'm sorry for, I can accept responsibility.

I've got a large heart.

I can seek assistance.

I am secure and well-cared for.

I have a lot to be thankful for.

I have faith in myself.

I still have so much more to learn about myself.

I have the ability to make a difference in people's lives.

I have no control over other people, but I do have power over how I respond to them.

I'm entertaining to be around.

I can let go of my problems and discover peace.

I am stunning.

When something bothers me, I can take good action.

I'm certain that everything will work out in the end.

I can find comedy in the mundane.

I may request the particular type of assistance I require.

When I'm bored or uninspired, I turn to my imagination.

I'm an excellent listener.

I have a pleasant personality.

I am aware of my inadequacies.

The opinions of others will not prevent me from being my true self.

When I'm feeling low, I can brighten myself up.

I can put myself in the shoes of others.

I adore myself completely.

My family adores me without reservation.

Today is a new day.

There is nothing I cannot accomplish.

I am capable of advocating for myself.

I'm going to accomplish a lot today.

MY EYES ENJOY SEX, AND THROUGH THEM I DO TOO

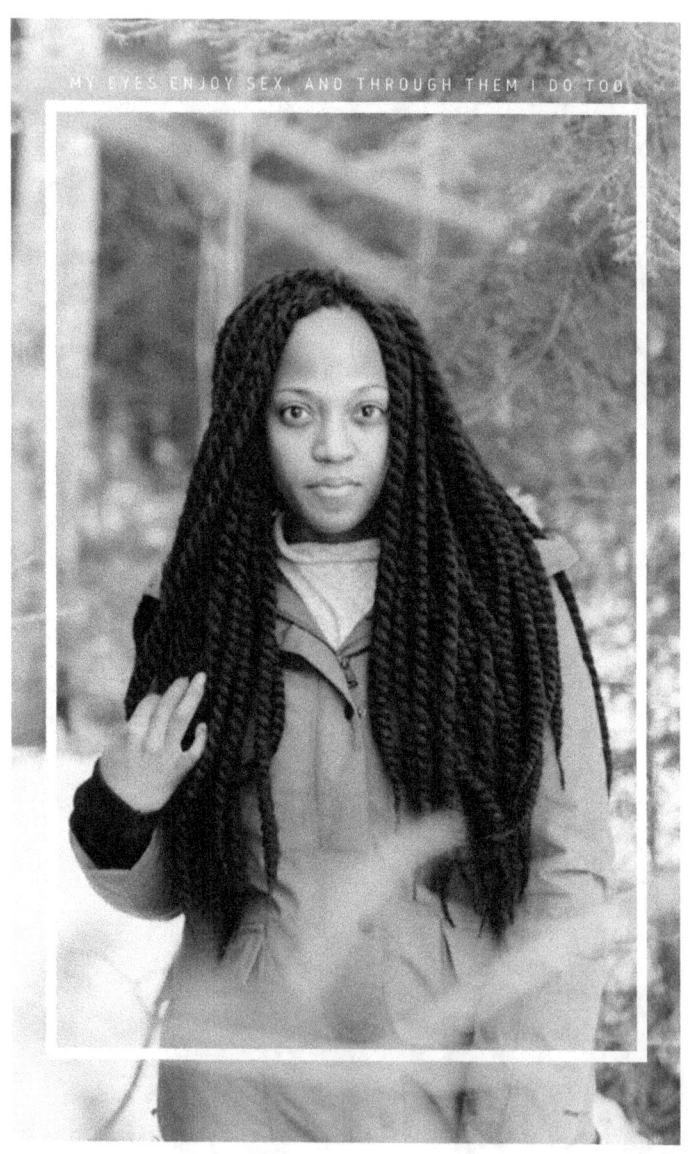

My thoughts are valuable.

I would want to have me as a friend.

It's fine to be unique.

When anything bothers me, I can talk to an adult.

When I'm upset, I can ask for a hug.

I have the ability to take the time necessary to comprehend my emotions.

I have a wide range of interests.

In truth, I have nothing to be embarrassed of.

I'm not embarrassed to weep.

I can unwind and be myself.

I have the option of surrounding myself with individuals that value me for who I am.

My body is something I love.

I am eager to learn from my friends and colleagues.

I look after my physical health because I adore myself.

I don't need to measure myself against others.

I will always give it my all.

I enjoy learning new things.

I'm precisely where I'm supposed to be.

I enjoy meeting new people.

I am a powerful person on the inside and out.

I am patient and composed.

Today is a lovely day.

Healing Trauma

Today, I chose myself.

I do not hold myself responsible for my childhood experiences/trauma.

I choose to create a peaceful and secure environment for myself.

I take full ownership of my mind, body, and soul.

Setting boundaries allows me to build safety in my life.

I replace hatred, wrath, and irritation with focused and pleasant connections with people.

Today, my interactions and decisions are surrounded by love and tranquility.

My traumatic/abusive experiences do not determine who I am as a person.

I let go of loneliness, feelings of guilt, hurt, humiliation, and replaced them with me, the black goddess who walks confidently, with aura radiating brilliantly.

I give myself permission to embrace nice words and ideas about myself.

Despite my anguish, I sincerely and deeply love and accept myself.

Today, I am comforting my inner kid.

My worth is equal to that of any other person.

My inner child is waiting to be recognized.

I easily accept love and kindness.

Setting hard limits is second nature to me.

Through my activities, I am ensuring that my inner child is secure from harm.

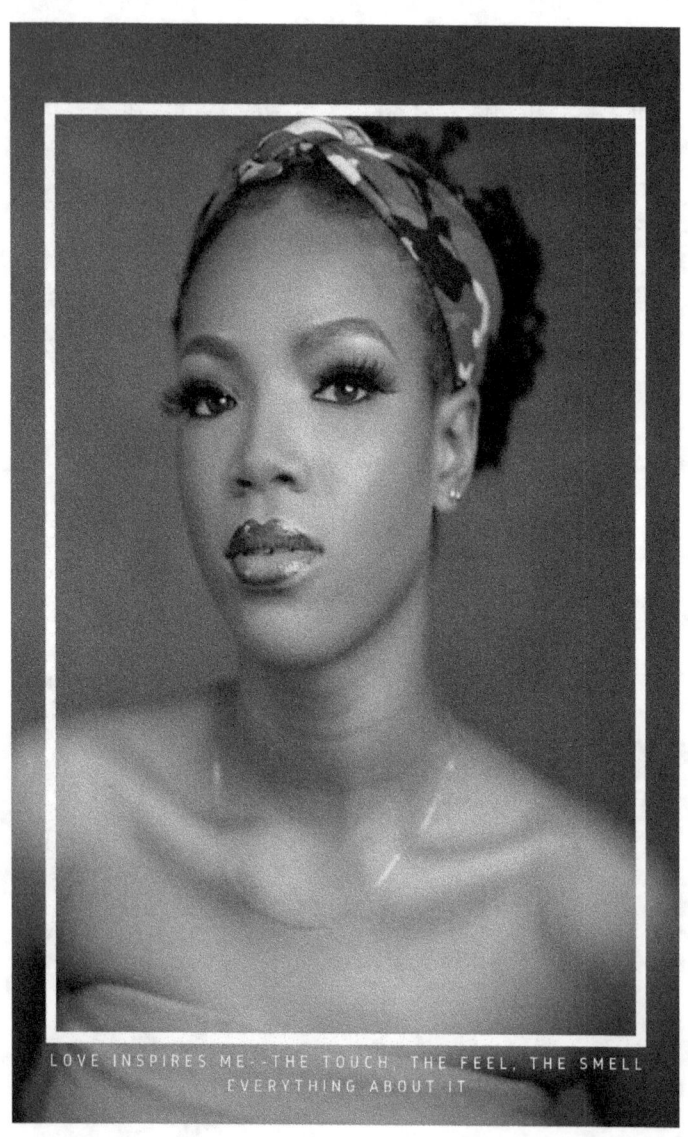

LOVE INSPIRES ME--THE TOUCH, THE FEEL, THE SMELL EVERYTHING ABOUT IT

I assure my inner child of his or her protection by speaking words of kindness, compassion, and hope to him or her.

My being is comforted by a sense of calm and tranquility.

My willingness to keep my vows reflects the significance of my self-connection.

I interrupt the pattern of thoughts and behaviors that leads to reliving the trauma.

I recognize and accept that healing is a possibility.

Conquering Goals

My relationship with myself as a black woman is of no greater importance to anyone but myself.

I'm getting better every day.

I am sufficient.

I am now a leader.

Every one of my problems has a solution.

When I face the difficulties of being a black woman, I persist in being myself, and continue to grow.

I forgive myself for my errors.

My errors assist me to learn and progress.

I'm perfect the way I am.

I am brave and self-assured.

Today is going to be an excellent day.

I have folks that adore and admire me.

I have power over my own happiness.

I am confident in my ambitions and dreams.

I fight for what I believe in.

Today, this river of positive thoughts flows through black women everywhere.

It's fine to not know everything.

I'm capable of overcoming any obstacle.

I have faith in myself and my ability.

I have the ability to make my dreams come true.

I am significant.

Good things are on their way to me.

Optimistic sentiments result from my positive thinking.

When I move outside of my comfort zone, my confidence develops.

I am open to new experiences and eager to learn.

Today, I'm going to face my anxieties.

I will get back up if I fall.

Each new day brings new bright stars to guide my spirit to new heights.

I only make comparisons with myself.

Each new day, I feel complete and secure in living a life of intention striving to reach my goals.

It is sufficient for me to do my best.

I'm capable of doing anything.

I can be anyone I want to be.

Chapter 8:

Affirmations to Perfect Your Self-Image

*Honor her for all that her hands have done,
and let her works bring her praise at the city gate.*

—Proverbs 31:31

This is a time to remember our self-image isn't defined by the prejudices of others, nor by how we esteem our sexy bodies. Through the scenes of our lives, as we envision our future, achieving our goals and fulfilling our hearts, our self-image is revealed through our actions as we better ourselves, earning self-respect, improving self-esteem, and raising our self-worth.

Affirming our self-image can be one of the strongest things we can do for our self-esteem. Not only should we say these affirmations out loud, but we should also believe them. Whenever we are going about our life, we need to recite them to ourselves in our

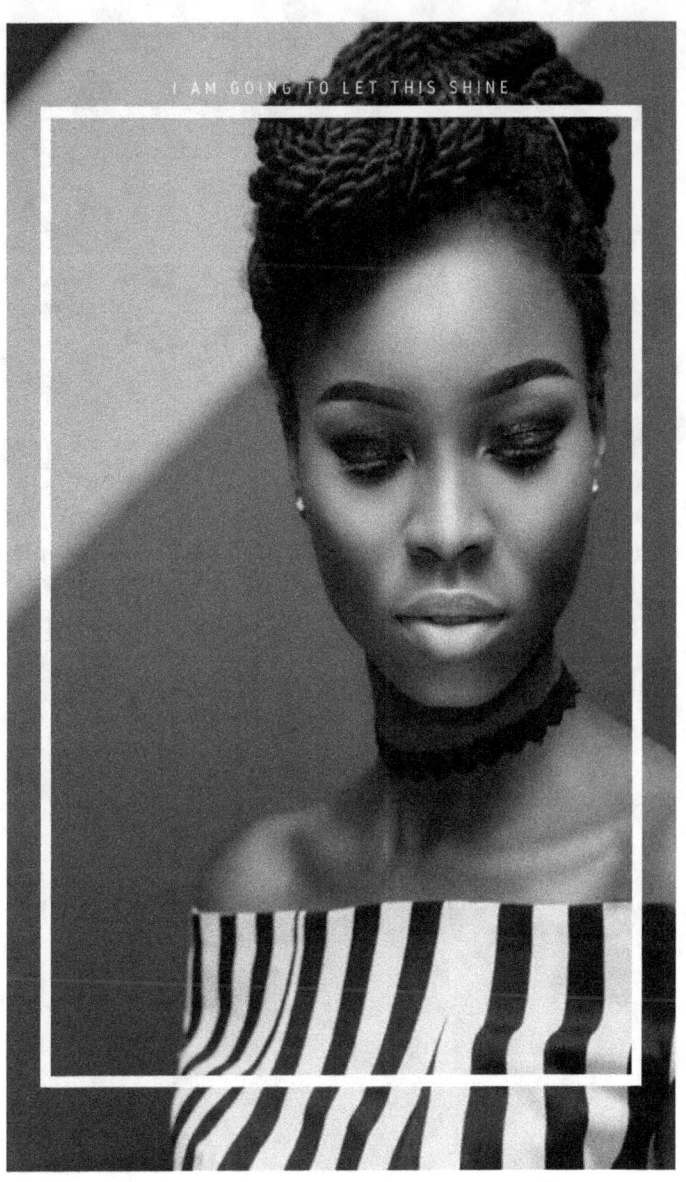

minds. There are various spheres of life that are affected by our self-image, namely:

- Our physical,
- mental,
- social,
- emotional,
- and spiritual well-being.

When we work hard to look our best, we achieve an overall improvement in many spheres of our lives. Our moods get better because our confidence rubs off on others. We are able to go out more and meet people, making significant connections. This is hard to come by when we are consumed with thoughts about whether we are living up to someone's standards – so we set our own! Our emotions, therefore, improve, as well as our overall ability to look into our spiritual lives.

I exude beauty, radiance, and elegance.

I communicate and connect with others using my gestures, movements, and my very presence, not just my words.

I adore myself. My heavenly Father created me in his image, and I am one-of-a-kind.

God loves me completely.

My confidence is skyrocketing as I recognize my own self-worth.

I feel I am deserving of love.

My body is in good shape, my intellect is sharp, and my spirit is at peace.

I'm bursting at the seams with energy and excitement.

I've been bestowed with a plethora of abilities, which I'm only getting started with.

I am stronger than bad ideas and deeds.

My fury is washed away by a flood of compassion, and it is replaced with love.

I forgive those who have wronged me in the past and remember to stand on my own foundation of integrity.

My life is increasing, growing, and prospering.

Creative energy rushes through me, causing me to come up with new and creative ideas.

I have the qualities required to be incredibly successful.

My capacity to overcome obstacles is endless, and my potential for success is limitless.

Happiness is an option. Today, I'm going to choose happiness.

I am brave and daring. I can stand up for myself.

I can accomplish all things through Christ, who gives me strength.

Today, I'm breaking old behaviors and forming new, more positive ones.

My thoughts are full of hope, and my life is full of abundance.

I am fortunate to have an amazing family and excellent friends.

I am adored and valued.

Everything that is happening right now is for my ultimate good.

I am at peace with everything that has occurred, is occurring, and will occur.

I am a fearfully and beautifully created being.

I forgive myself for my faults and shortcomings in the past.

I AM THE NURTURER OF MY HEART

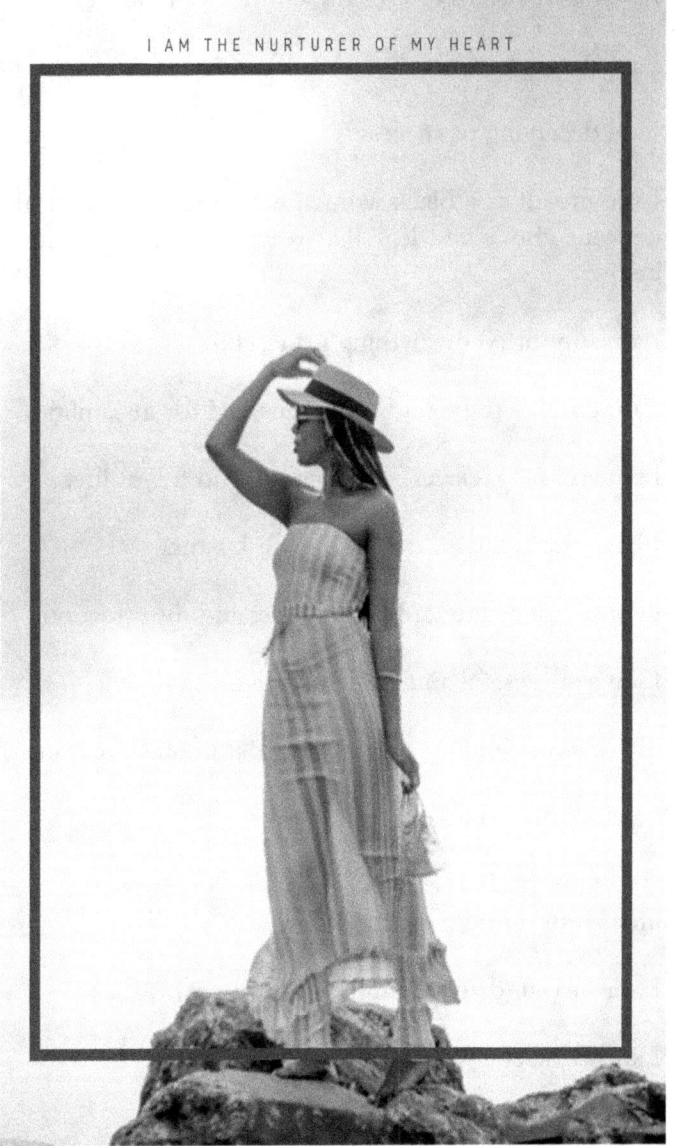

Every day, I learn to love myself more and more.

I am deserving of love.

I am deserving of success.

I see myself as a black woman with arms that reach the heavens above and legs that reach deep into the roots below.

I am supported in anything I do in life.

I am entitled to be fairly compensated for my abilities.

I am stunning, clever, entertaining, and full of life.

I have the ability to design the life I want.

People respect my effort, my time, and my affection.

I am a successful and content individual.

[fill in your name] is one of my most impressive traits.

I have faith in myself.

What my goals mean to me is what is important—my life is mine and I'm living it now.

I am surrounded by kindness and optimism.

I am sufficient.

People want to know what I think and what I believe. My opinion matters.

I'm perfect the way I am.

My self-love is mirrored in every aspect of my life.

I value myself, and others do as well.

Everything I desire in life is within my grasp.

There's nothing I can't get my hands on.

Wonderful things come into my life.

I'm doing a fantastic job.

There is nothing I need to do or be in order to deserve love or respect.

I am entire and whole.

For me, anything is possible.

My physique is lovely just the way it is.

What I desire is on its way to me.

I have everything I require to be successful.

My efforts are recognized and acknowledged.

I am deserving of the accolades I have received.

I am equally as valuable as anybody else.

I deserve to be loved, to be happy, and to have fun in my life.

I feel I have a promising future ahead of me.

I'm a good employee, and I deserve some time off to unwind.

I am grateful for my history, content with my present, and excited about my future.

I am grateful for my physique and enjoy the way it appears.

I am surrounded by people I adore, and they adore me in return.

When I want to, I can and should say "no" without hesitation.

I am not required to perform all that people ask of me.

I have the right to my own viewpoint, which does not have to coincide with anyone else's.

I am a nice person, and there is no need for me to prove that to anyone.

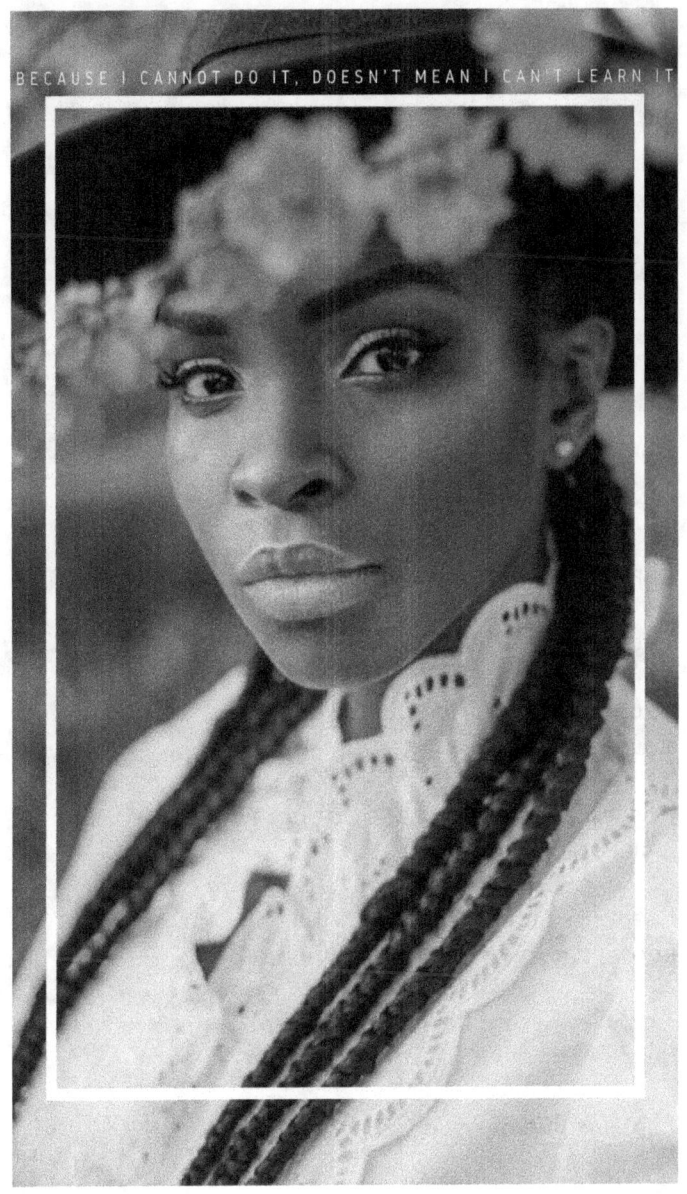

Regardless of what others think, I am gorgeous with all of my distinct characteristics.

My pals realize that I am a fantastic friend.

I am at peace with my failings and faults in the past.

I am entitled to enjoy myself in life.

I feel at ease in my own body and thinking.

I am capable of big things and have the strength, resources, and talents to accomplish my objectives.

I accept myself and everyone else.

I have a fantastic life full of experiences.

Every day, I grow as a person.

Every day, I learn and improve as I adjust to new situations.

I never stop learning, both from my own and from the faults of others.

People enjoy chatting with me because I am knowledgeable and entertaining.

The world is a wonderful place, and I am grateful to be here today.

I am absolutely loved.

When I sense injustice, I have the right to speak up.

Even though my contributions are minor, they make a significant difference in the world.

I forgive myself and anyone who has harmed me.

Every day, I endeavor to do my best, and that is sufficient.

I am a caring person that cares about other people.

My best buddy is myself.

Every day, I learn to love myself more.

In whatever I do, I have the support of my family and friends.

My point of view is valuable, and people actually care about it.

I am unstoppable in the pursuit of my objectives.

I am gorgeous in my own right, and I don't need to compare myself to anyone else.

I am worthy, and my value is unaffected by the opinions of others.

I am unique in my own right, and I don't need to act like someone else to impress others.

Every day, I move closer to my goals.

I am imaginative and have original ideas. My effort deserves to be recognized.

I am a strong person who can defend myself and others when necessary.

I am unique, and no one can replace me.

Nature has blessed me with my beauty, knowledge, and abilities, and I am grateful.

I have earned the right to prioritize myself over everyone else.

Chapter 9:

Affirmations to Ignite the Power of Sex

Let him kiss me with the kisses of his mouth—for your love is more delightful than wine.

—Song of Solomon 1:2

Let's have an honest conversation about our sex lives. We could use a scale from 1 to 10, where we gauge our satisfaction level; 10 being very satisfied, 1 not at all. But let's just slow it down—is sex just for satisfaction? Or is there something else? Black women like you and me are about to break down the taboo subject of this amazingly beautiful union. Maybe it's a chore? We'll be thrilled. Maybe it's an unknown? We'll explore it with openness. Maybe the heat is already up? Let's reveal the secrets.

Now, before going and having sex with just anyone, we can't just justify it with science and health alone. Oh my dear, no! Love is the emotion we need to find—love for our pretty black selves. As well, we should know how to trust a person and communicate well with them before letting them become a permanent fixture in our lives. When a man knows how to please us, and it feels right, there are many ways to give signs and signals of just how much we enjoy it. Beyond that, the harmony which results can be just amazing.

First, and I know you're all passionate to read this, there are various reasons why sex is good for us, besides it being delightfully pleasurable. Here are the reasons:

- Lowers blood pressure
- Boosts immune system
- Lowers the risk of heart disease
- Increases dopamine

I'm proud of my sexuality and sensuality.

I'm thankful for my body and the incredible sexual pleasure it gives me.

In and out of the bedroom, I am appealing, fun, and seductive. I drive my partner insane.

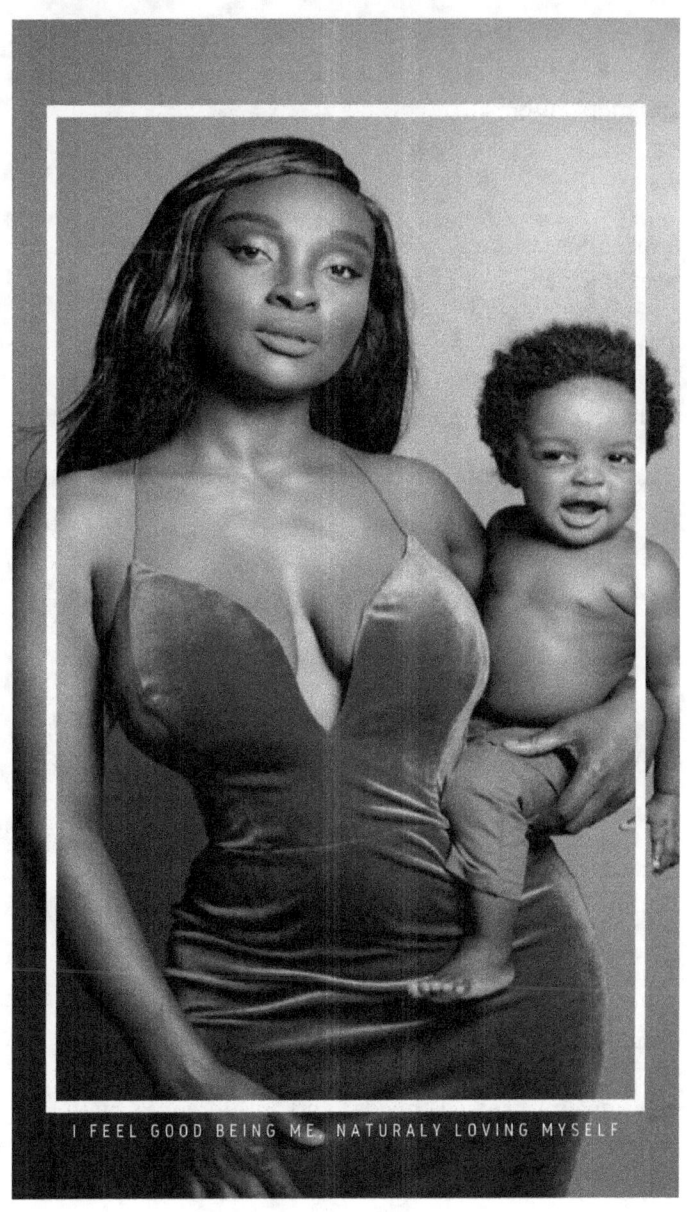

Every pore on my body exudes confidence. My sweetheart is drawn to me because I exude a dazzling, magnetic aura.

I have earned the right to be happy.

I am a sexual deity. For the partner and me, I pick sex as a spiritual, soulful energy exchange.

I am unstoppable.

I am free and secure to pursue my sexual urges.

Sexually and emotionally, I am secure. I have faith in my capacity to select worthy sexual partners and form meaningful bonds.

My body needs to be cherished, appreciated and cared for.

I believe in my intuition. I have every ability and technique I could possibly require. I'm comfortable in bed and am continuously looking to improve.

Sexual arousal is a pleasurable experience. In the bedroom, I am daring, at ease, and self-assured.

I feel liberated, full, and finished.

I take care of my sexual and emotional needs.

Sharing my sexual needs and preferences with my partner makes me feel at ease and protected.

I am entitled to a fulfilling and passionate sexual life.

I am deserving of all the closeness, pleasure, romance, and sexual connection I seek.

My libido has sprung to life.

I know how to enjoy myself as well as delight my partner. It's something I'm naturally good at.

I value closeness and respect limits. My relationship is visible and audible to me. They notice and hear me.

I am brimming with orgasmic, sensuous, sexual energy.

My sex life is flourishing. Sexually, I am full and satisfied.

My spouse and I approach sex as a holy environment with dignity and respect.

I am totally there in the bedroom, tuned in to all of the feelings accessible to me in my sexual encounters.

Every sexual contact is distinct, one-of-a-kind, and exhilarating. I am as sexually daring as I want to be.

My bedroom is a secure haven of calm, independence, and sexual fulfillment.

I'm overwhelmed with love and thankfulness.

My body is in good health and works well to offer and receive pleasure.

My sex life is consistent and enjoyable.

I pay attention to my body's demands and gently lead my partner to meet them.

I am open-minded and eager to try new things in bed.

My sexual life is crucial to my health and stress alleviation; therefore, I prioritize it.

I'm sexually appealing and forceful.

To attain sexual well-being, I study my body with curiosity.

Rejection from a possible partner has no effect on me.

I regularly have strong peaks that please both my mind and body.

I am a seductive and appealing woman/man. When I feel it, others notice it as well.

My bed is a haven where I feel cherished, safe, and content.

In my sexual life, I am always at ease and confident.

I can be honest with my lover about what I like and dislike.

In bed, I can be anybody I want, and I enjoy experimenting.

I can open out to my spouse about my anxieties and insecurities.

I know what I want, and I get it on a regular basis.

My sex life is thrilling and enjoyable.

I'm sexy, and I'm aware of it!

I am entitled to sexual pleasure on a regular basis.

I feel alive when I have moments of pleasure.

I am naturally leading my lover to give me the utmost pleasure.

I can really unwind and enjoy the experience.

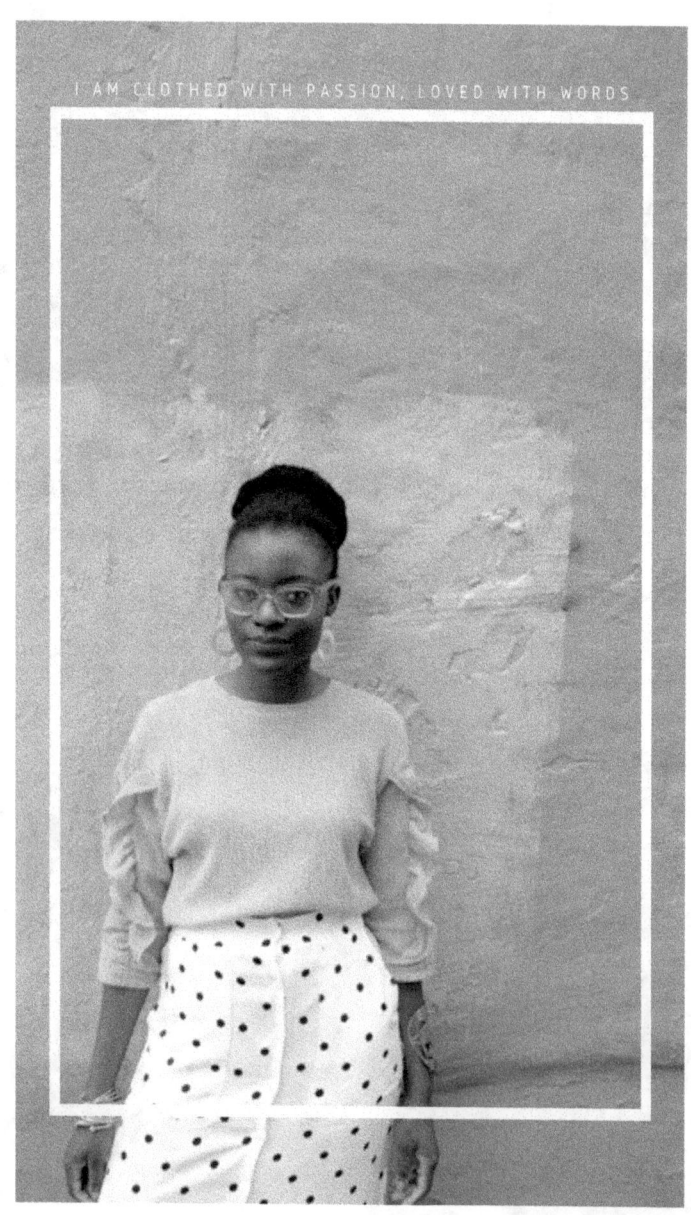

I only date people that are kind and considerate.

My eyes have a magnetic pull.

I am a sexual attraction expert.

My sexual orientation attracts partners that are a great match for me.

I effortlessly grab attention and curiosity.

My sexuality is addicting, and my lover is always looking for more.

Potential partners think I'm sexy and beautiful.

I'm proud of my sexuality and sensuality.

I only pursue passionate relationships with clear limits.

Every time my partner sees me, he or she turns on.

In bed, I feel crazy and drive my lover insane.

In bed, I may be a tiger or a kitten, and my conduct is both natural and adaptable.

I make the process of mutual sexual arousal enjoyable and simple.

If they knew about my sexual adventures, they'd be jealous.

I never allow my sexual life to become dull or routine; I enjoy surprises and new experiences.

My sex life is fantastic and fulfilling.

I'm buzzing with good sexual energy and attracting more of it.

I'm brimming with natural sexual vigor.

I am deserving of a kind and caring companion.

I attract the right companion, and he or she can't get enough of me.

I am attractive and always catch my selected partner's attention.

With my sexual enthusiasm, I continue to attract hot partners.

I'm thankful for my attractive physique and all of the sexual pleasure it provides.

My body is a sanctuary, and every one of my partners regards it as such.

Conclusion

If you have read this multiple times, bravo. I say, read it again and again. Breathe a sigh of relief; you know you have now sparked an incredible passion within yourself with this three-part formula. A perfect child image for yourself, ready to be born again through sex. Ladies, please take time to think through the journey you took in this book. Small and short as it was, the few minutes it took to read it will affect your life in marvelous ways. Different affirmations may become more relevant to you through various stages of your life—so keep it closer than you might think.

We know the majesty of the woman that we all want to be. Well, maybe we don't know everything yet; we might need another month or year. Regardless, reading through this book and series should help us understand where we could go with our next steps. The depths of being a black woman are truly great. We are incomparable in the ways through which we express our beauty. So, we don't have to copy someone else—we can be ourselves. We don't have to feel like we are lacking in our femininity. With these affirmations, we are igniting the fire within us that directs us where we need to go.

We can start making affirmation mornings a ritual. After choosing the affirmations we would like to work on, we can wake up 5 minutes earlier and say them out loud before going about our day. This might sound like a tedious task, but life is really what we make of it. So, if we put in the effort we need to put in, we will reap a great harvest in return. After all, we don't want life to just happen to us. Instead, let's take ownership of what we will allow into our lives and live our destinies.

I believe that the power we have as women is in our community. When we stick hand in hand, we will be able to help each other face the biggest challenges. When you find that this book has helped you in any way, spread the word with your friends and family. Don't underestimate the impact you could have on those around you. By radiating love, you get from your self-awareness, you will lead women to ask themselves how you got that radiance you emit. Take that opportunity to tell them how you got a closer look inside yourself with this book. And leave us a 5-star review on Amazon to help others.

Life is hard, and well, as black women the best thing we can do for ourselves is stand together throughout our trials. When we do this, we conquer anything formed against us and bust through walls meant to hold us back.

Welcome the Nature of Mothers, Nurture the Innocence of Daughters, and Manifest the Career of Your Dreams

Introduction

If you are reading this book, I believe that you can agree that the plight of the black woman is one that is often overlooked. Many can say that it is hard to be a black person in society. But I believe that it is even worse to be a black woman. You see, black women are the ones who often carry the burdens of their communities on their shoulders. If you think long enough, I am sure you can list the names of black women you have encountered in life who went above and beyond to restore the damage of social ills in our communities.

With the rise in teenage pregnancy and drug abuse, black women are left in a very fragile place. I wrote this book series for women because I believe that there is very little that motivates the black woman to go above the situation she faces at home. I chose this demographic of people specifically because I believe the old saying that when you teach a girl child, you teach a community.

With so many distractions and stressors in black communities, it becomes hard for black mothers to feel safe in their maternity. In this book in particular, I write about affirmations to welcome the nature of mothers. Motherhood is a very strong force that can be diverted with time. Some black women find themselves in abusive households where they hardly think through. These situations can severely pacify our maternity. They can create in us hardened hearts. Whereas we have to be loving and gentle to nurture our children, we can instead be hard and cold. I hope you enjoy chapter one as much as I enjoyed writing it for you.

The second chapter travels down from the mother to the daughter. Our children imitate everything that we do. They criticize each of our actions and they will choose to emulate behaviors in us that they like. Sometimes these behaviors are not healthy behaviors. You see, once we become mothers, we need to find it in ourselves to give and still be able to grow in our own skin. If you have a daughter who has had to grow up a little too fast, her innocence may have been broken. Children who experience situations where they have to take care of their younger siblings at an early age tend to forget that they too are children who can remain gentle and fragile. Chapter two is dedicated to these girls who would like to reconnect with their child-like innocence.

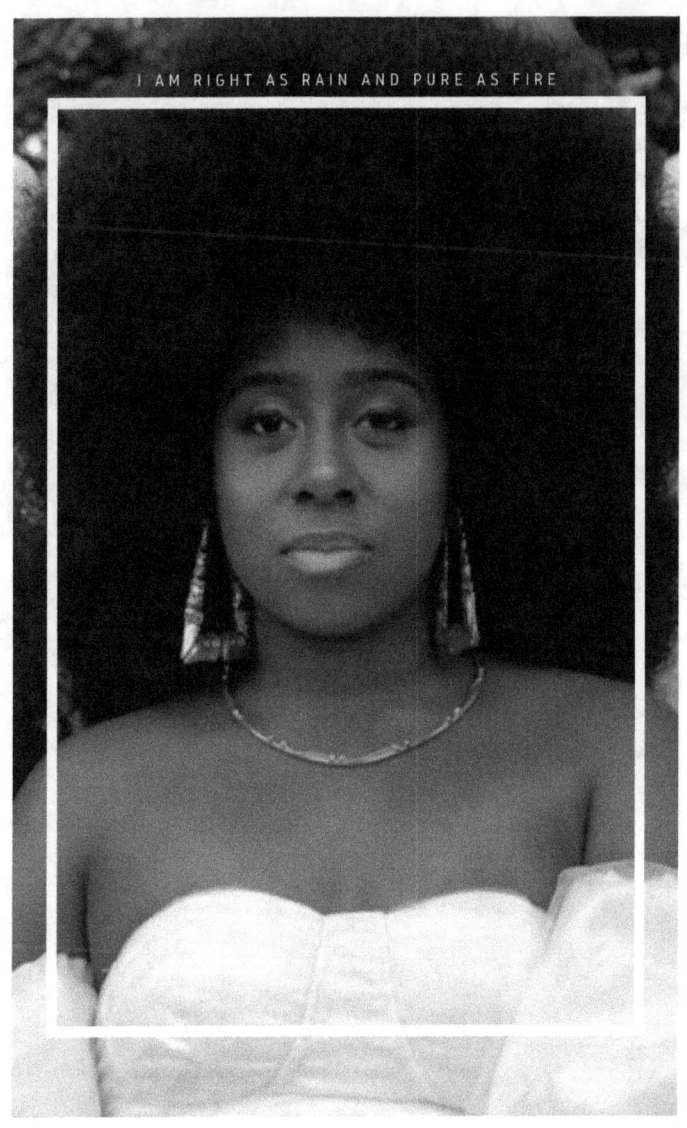

Finally, the third chapter is dedicated to all black women who want to get ahead in life. I believe that every black woman needs to acquire some kind of financial independence. We are all good at different things. Once you know what you are good at, you can be in a better position to capitalize on that skill. If you had dreams of opening a business or going to school, use the affirmations in this chapter to help you gather confidence in yourself and your skill. You do not need to have an idea that already exists in the market, nor should your business idea land you millions of dollars. But if you can work with your hands, employ a few other women, and provide for your family, you will have gone above and beyond. So what are you waiting for? Go for it!

Chapter 10:

Affirmations to Welcome the Nature of Mothers

"These commandments that I give you today are to be on your hearts. Impress them on your children. Talk about them when you sit at home and when you walk along the road, when you lie down and when you get up."

–Deuteronomy 6:6-7

Crystal: **Lapis Lazuli** to feel calm amidst Mother Nature

We can all agree that mothers are the pillars of our society. A mother's love is not only nurturing, but it is also healing. When a child is hurt, they can easily forget the pain when they find themselves back in their mother's arms. That said, it can be quite hard to understand how you need to mother. The fabric of gender roles has become so imbalanced that black mothers tend to do everything in the household. As a result, you may just be an exhausted mother. You may fail to spend time with your children. Maybe you have lost touch with who they are becoming and your influence on them has thinned. I completely understand.

The following affirmations were created for a situation like yours. They were also created for other cases where black mothers want to touch base with their maternal instinct. What I can tell you is that you need not be hard on yourself. Yes, a lot rests on your shoulders, but you don't have to go on this journey alone. And if you equip yourself with all the information you need, you will make far fewer mistakes. But in any case, the best advice I can give you is to mother from a place of love and all will be fine.

Are you a black mother trying to reconnect with your maternal instincts? Do you feel like you could be doing more as a mother for your children and family? Then I am glad to have you here.

For those listening, follow the prompts. If you are reading, remember to repeat these affirmations not just mentally, but with your voice. You can do it, girl; this is a profound change! The world is waiting and you have the power! Use your voice and believe in what makes you ultimately powerful—your voice and your projections of fire!

There is no such thing as a perfect mother, but there are a million ways to be a good one.

My children consider me a blessing.

Only I can provide my children with a contented mother.

The love of a mother liberates.

I'm doing an excellent job.

I can rely on my maternal instincts.

My child will be my lifetime teacher.

With each new day, I learn to be a better mother.

Today, I'm going to focus on the wonderful elements of parenthood.

Motherly love is the fuel that allows a normal human being to accomplish the impossible.

In order to be a good mother, I will take care of myself.

Motherhood is more powerful than natural laws.

It's a distinct joy to be able to participate in creation.

I'm doing everything I can for my children, and it's enough.

I am grateful for my power to bring life into the world.

Being a mother teaches you about strengths you didn't know you have and how to deal with anxieties you didn't know you had.

I am just what my child requires.

I am the most influential person in my child's life.

With each passing day, I become a more confident mother.

I am providing the finest possible future for my children.

Motherhood is where all love begins and ends.

We may discover that by giving birth to our children, we are giving life to new possibilities inside ourselves.

I deserve some downtime.

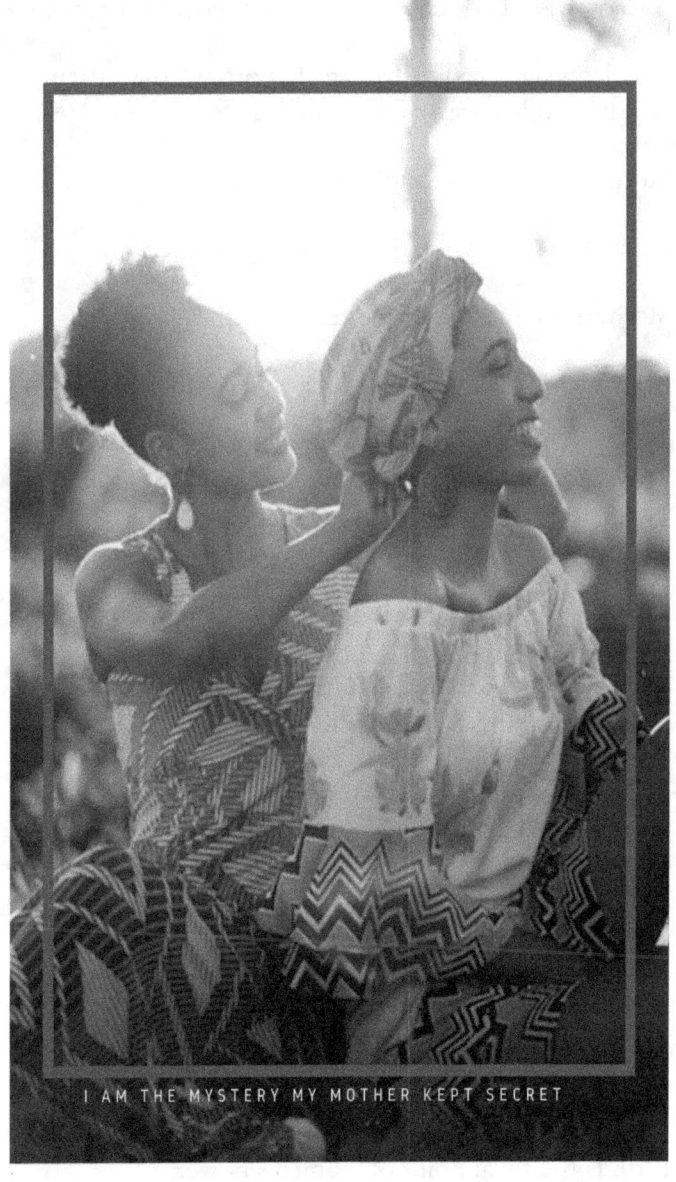

As a mother, I am deserving of the accolades I receive.

No language can adequately portray the strength, beauty, and heroism of a mother's love.

Motherhood has highlighted my talents.

I am an excellent role model for my children.

Motherhood has made me feel attractive.

I can accomplish anything because I'm a mother.

Today, I'm going to laugh with my kids.

Today, I will refrain from passing judgment.

I'm not going to sweat the minor stuff today.

My children are unconcerned with my imperfections.

There is no impact more potent than a mothers.

I'm not going to dwell on my fears today.

I don't expect to be an ideal mother.

Today I have enough patience for my children.

Motherhood is a never-ending act of optimism.

I'm making wonderful, life-long memories with my kids.

Birth is the focal point of women's power.

I know better than anybody what my children require.

I have sentiments that should be acknowledged.

I make a difference in the lives of my family members.

My child is just fine the way he or she is.

My faults from yesterday are unimportant.

As a mother, I have the right to seek assistance.

A mother is a lady who sees the light when you only see darkness.

My family believes in me.

Every day, I learn with my child.

I am thankful for the chance to raise my child.

The difficulties I confront make me a better mommy.

In my family's life, I maintain order.

Everything will be alright in the end.

I'm growing better and better every day.

I'm not a horrible mother. I am a decent mother who is simply having a terrible day.

Simply take a big breath. This, too, will pass.

I'll try my best with the talents and tools I have.

Everything has its time and place.

I shall not be frightened or ashamed to seek such assistance.

When I need assistance, I will accept it.

Each dawn ushers in a new day. I'll do better next time. I can always get back up and try again.

I can accomplish almost everything, but not everything.

There is no one way to be a wonderful mother.

I will let go of my perfectionist standards and allow things to happen as they will.

Even when things appear to be hectic, there is serenity and love in my household.

I am the perfect mom for my child to develop and succeed in life.

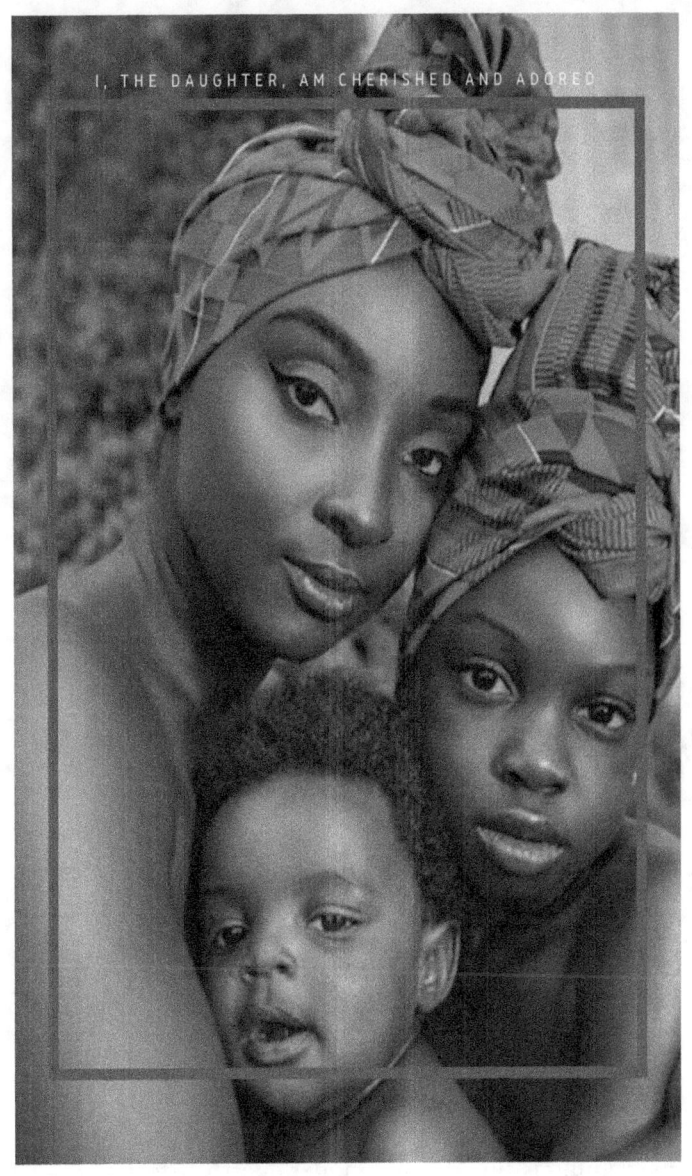

Everything I do is for the benefit of my family.

I am confident in my ability. I know a lot more than I think.

I'm going to talk to myself like I'm talking to someone I care about.

I accept myself precisely as I am and will no longer demand perfection from myself in order to love myself.

I am capable of incredible things if I believe it and act with meaning and purpose.

I am eager to study because I believe that the more I learn, the more I will grow.

I trust my instincts and believe that nothing will be thrown at me that I cannot manage.

I have boundless potential. I was designed for more.

Only I have power over my ideas and actions.

My heart is wide open. I am ready to forgive and begin afresh.

My youngsters have boundless potential. They, too, are built for more.

Even in the midst of a hurricane, I have the fortitude to stay calm.

Everything is fine. I can conquer every obstacle.

I have the ability to effect change.

Today, I've decided to be at peace.

I have control over how I feel today.

I have the ability to choose.

I'm proud of myself and what I've done.

I can't alter people; therefore I'll accept them as they are.

I'm thankful to be alive. Life is really valuable.

Negative ideas and habits are no longer serving me, therefore I let them go.

I have plenty of options, and possibilities abound.

It makes no difference what other people say or do. I make the decision to make positive changes in my life.

Every difficulty is a blessing.

I choose faith over dread.

All of my issues have solutions. Rather than focusing on the problem, I envision solutions.

It's fine if I make a mistake. Everyone makes errors. It is a necessary component of the learning process.

Chapter 11:

Affirmations to Nurture the Innocence of Daughters

"The Lord bless you, my daughter," he replied. "This kindness is greater than that which you showed earlier: You have not run after the younger men, whether rich or poor."

–Ruth 3:10

Crystal: **Rhodochrosite** to faithfully inspire compassion for ourselves.

Before we were women, we were girls. We were girls filled with so many dreams and ambitions. One other thing we had was innocence. What is child-like innocence, you may ask? Children are innocent because they lack the ability to reason the way adults do. This often leads to them making a lot of mistakes. They are trusting, honest, and generally kind. These are qualities that help them explore the world in the

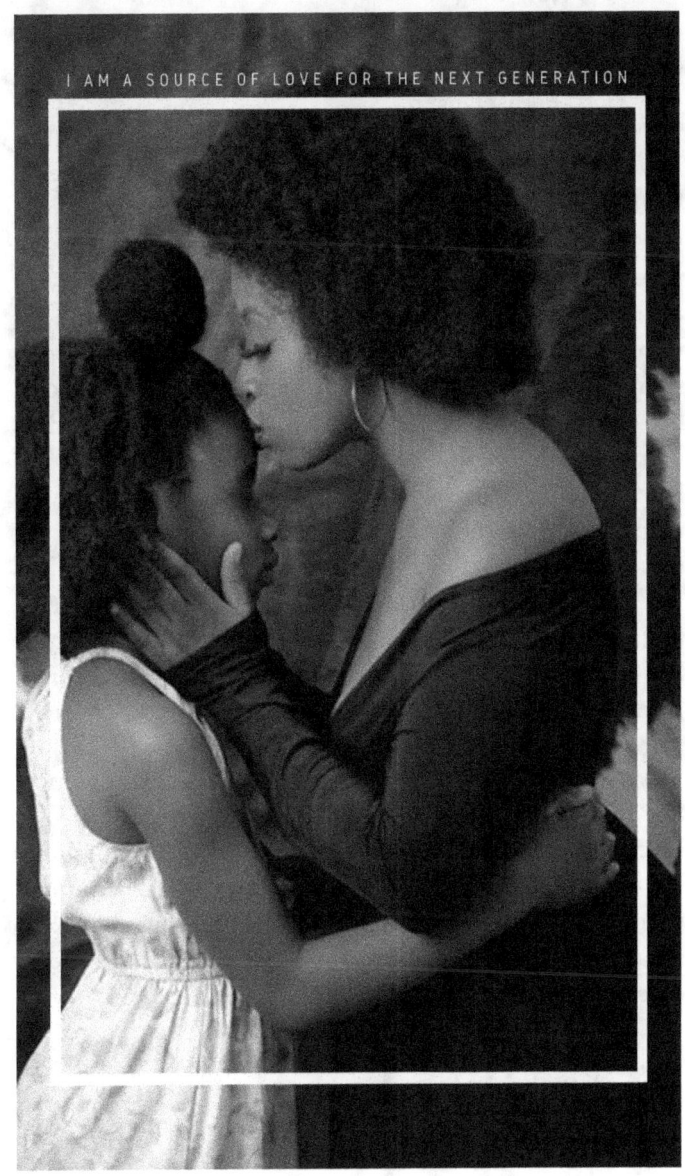

early stages of life. Their ability to trust adults and their environments helps them form an idea of the world they find themselves in.

It is a sad realization that not all girls have this privilege. With this innocence comes the fragility and vulnerability of children. So, although as mothers we would like to protect our children at all times, there are times when they are hurt in this world. Life is unpredictable. I had a friend who had to leave and work in another country for a while before she could move her family there. She had three daughters, the oldest being 14 years old. As a caring mother she arranged for her sister to stay with the kids, but the sister was neglectful. The oldest daughter then felt she had to try to make sure that things carried on the way they did when her mother was around. I remember my friend telling me when she came back that her eldest daughter has not been the same since. It was as though she grew three years older in just three months.

You see, children know nothing about their innocence. So, they don't know that it has to be protected. As a black mother you will notice changes in your daughter's development. These changes should cue what you need to do. I am glad that you have found this book. It means that you understand the importance of taking care of our femininity as black women.

I admire my childish naivety.

I unconditionally love my inner child.

I validate the ideas and feelings of my inner child.

I pay attention to the demands of my inner child.

With love, understanding, and compassion, I re-parent my inner child.

I have faith in my inner kid.

My inner kid frequently knows the correct solution for me.

In the future, I plan to pay more attention to my inner kid.

Being naïve and vulnerable makes me feel protected.

I've decided to embrace my inner child.

I'm going to quit neglecting my inner kid and start paying more attention to it.

It is okay to have different feelings than others.

It is okay to hold opposing views.

My inner kid deserves to be heard.

I am a brave person for revealing my weakness.

Today is the day for transformation.

I am brimming with energy and hope. I'm ready to discover happiness.

Many abilities have been bestowed to me. I'll put them to use today.

I am capable of overcoming bad ideas and events. I choose to be optimistic!

I am valuable.

I have the attributes required for success.

I am brave and I advocate for myself.

I will be there. I'll be optimistic.

I'll respect my need for rest and recharge.

I'm grateful for fresh experiences today.

Today, I embrace my finest self.

Today, I'm going to make an effort to locate some "me" time.

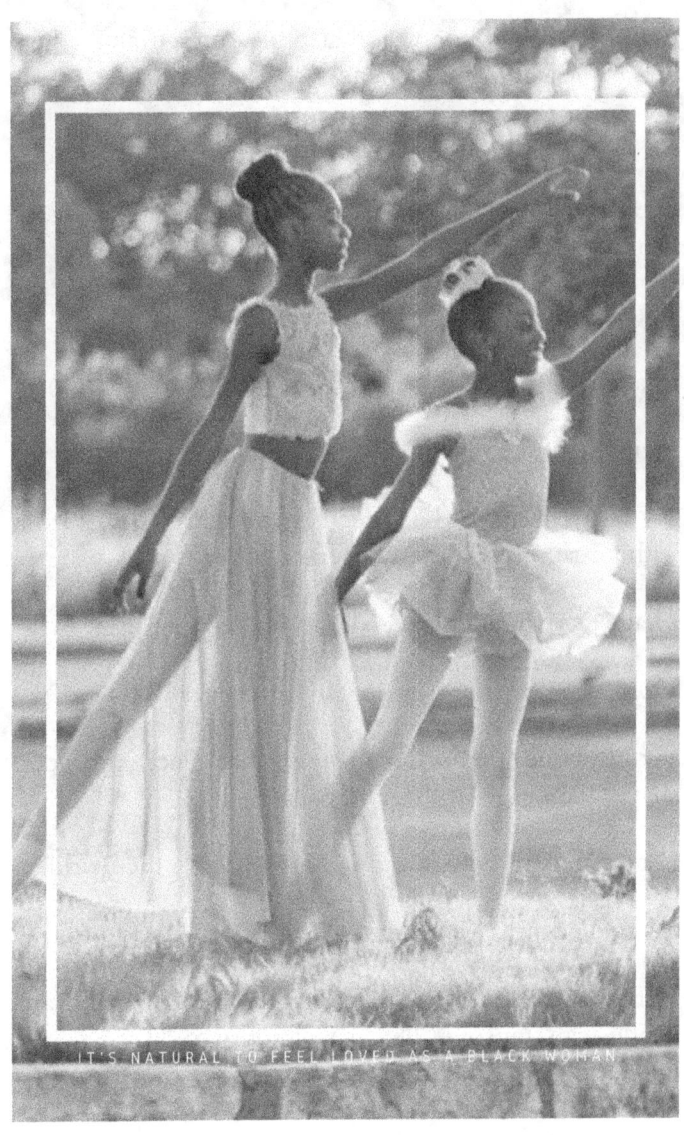

I choose to live in a way that brings myself and others peace, pleasure, and happiness.

I keep going. I am unyielding. I continue.

I've decided to let go of the past. My new road is in front of me. My new life begins now!

Today is the start of everything I desire.

I have replaced all of my negative ideas with good ones.

I am cheerful, radiant, and in good health.

My body needs to be cared for; therefore I nurture it with nutritious foods and energetic exercise.

I have enough energy for all of my everyday tasks.

I have a lot of energy, vigor, and happiness.

My physique is in good shape. My intellect is in good shape. I am eager to begin the day!

I enjoy making others smile; it is my gift to the world.

I exude positivity and vigor.

Times may be harsh, but they are only temporary. Things can improve. Things will improve.

I'm not going to worry about tomorrow. First and foremost, I shall enjoy the day ahead of me.

I have the ability to alter my story.

Challenges make us stronger and more resilient.

I choose optimism. I'd rather be happy. Both are all around me.

I've decided to face this task with grace and optimism.

I fully adore and embrace my figure.

I'm glad for the lessons I'll be learning today. I am glad for the opportunity to master new talents.

My child is developing normally.

My child is secure and cherished.

Every day, I make time for myself.

I am capable of overcoming any obstacles that may arise.

I am fully prepared for any circumstance.

I like and respect myself.

It's only a phase. It'll pass.

My baby is counting on me to be strong and fearless.

My personal needs are as important as my children's.

I'm in love with myself. I forgive myself and others when I make a mistake.

I am the perfect mom for my child, so I don't need to compare myself to others.

To make conscious parenting choices and decisions, I rely on my instincts.

Today, I'm going to focus on the wonderful elements of parenthood.

With each passing day, I am becoming a better mother.

I deserve to take care of myself and may respond to my emotional, physical, and spiritual needs without feeling guilty or apologetic.

I will let go of how I expect today to happen and welcome it with grace and joy.

I need to recognize myself for the work I accomplish every day.

I'm doing everything I can.

I am a patient person. I am physically present. I am optimistic.

What I do requires a really strong person and I should be proud of myself.

Finding new methods to eat healthily empowers me and puts me in charge.

I enjoy feeling powerful and fit. To feed my body, I choose to eat healthy and exercise consistently.

Every minute of the day, I accept bliss.

I'm going to make the remainder of my life the finest it can possibly be.

My enjoyment stems from inside.

I am deserving of happiness.

There are so many good things in my life.

I generate my pleasure by unconditionally loving every aspect of myself.

Today I'm feeling upbeat. I intend to share my joy with others.

Everything I do will bring me delight.

I was born to have a joyful life.

Following my delight shows me the way to my best existence.

Everything I attract reflects my happiness back to me.

I am willing to look for happiness in every moment.

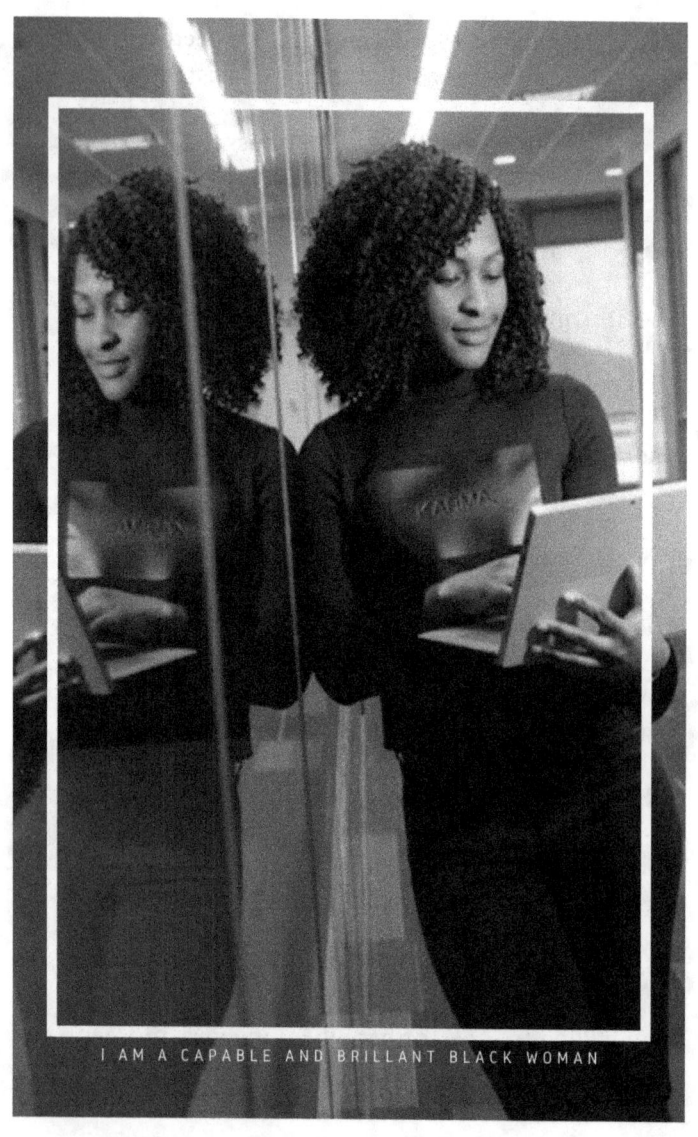

Chapter 12:

Affirmations to Manifest the Career of Your Dreams

"Submit to God and be at peace with Him;

in this way prosperity will come to you."

—Job 2:21

Crystal: **Peridot** to provide confidence for career decisions.

Think about your ambitions for a little while. Maybe you don't have many ambitions at the moment. Then, ask yourself what your ambitions were in the past. You see, different women live different lives. Sometimes the dreams we had when we were little honestly cannot go anywhere due to your present circumstances. So, many of us have to admit that ambitions are different for different women. Some black women may want a corner office in a big multimillion dollar company. But others may just want to see their small business succeed. There is also a group of black women who would rather like to see themselves build their family's strength and help their spouses with the family business. All are good ambitions.

Whatever your ambition may be, it can be quite hard to keep the wheels rolling. Some dreams require you to knock on several doors, and some doors will definitely not open. Some will open and see you out, but there are others that will open and offer you a seat inside. You need to be able to go through all the other doors that hit your face with grace, and this can be a hard task to expect from someone. So, the following affirmations are a great addition when you are not feeling your best confidence. Put a few of your favorites on your office wall or your fridge notebook.

Perhaps you, like many people, have a morning routine. Affirmations can be worked into that. Whether you do yoga in the morning or you sit to read a book, try to include a few of your favorite goal-specific affirmations into your routine.

My fantasies quickly become reality.

The future I desire is already taking shape.

I am drawing the things I desire into my life.

My ambitions are being realized.

My aspirations and objectives are drawn to me like a magnet.

Every day, good things happen in my life.

I live in a fantastic house in a fantastic neighborhood.

My life is full of love and pleasure.

Everything I do is a success.

New sums of money have appeared in my life.

I am in good health and full of positive energy.

I have a surplus of money.

Every day, I manifest more money.

I am willing to accept financial riches.

In my life, wealth and success are manifesting.

I am an abundance magnet.

I allow myself to be aligned with riches.

Money is continually entering my bank account.

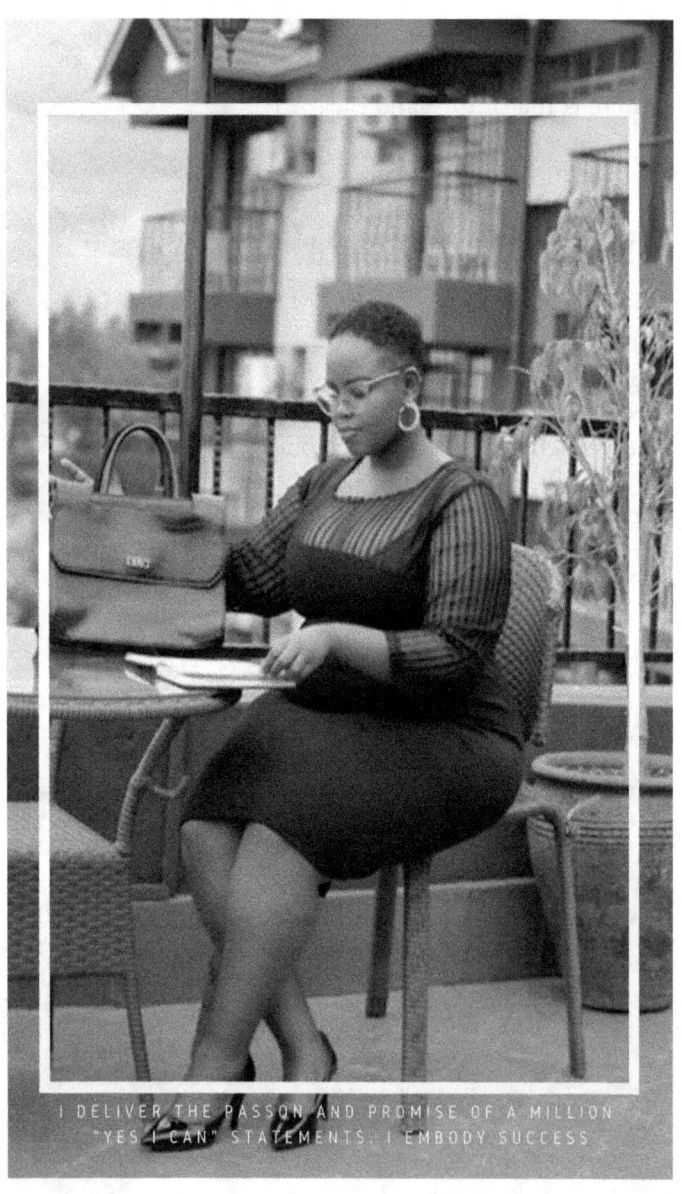

I DELIVER THE PASSION AND PROMISE OF A MILLION "YES I CAN" STATEMENTS. I EMBODY SUCCESS

My company is gaining a lot of paying clients.

I am a prosperous person.

My ideal job is becoming available to me.

I'm drawing my ideal job to myself.

The Universe is sending the perfect job for me.

Job offers are coming in thick and fast.

The Universe is bringing me a fantastic job.

I'm working at my ideal job and loving every minute of it.

I am obtaining an excellent job because I deserve it.

I have rewarding work that pays well.

I attract a prosperous career.

My good mindset is leading to new opportunities for me.

I'll get my dream job.

I'm having a lot of fun manifesting my dream job.

I am a self-assured and capable individual.

I have the qualifications for my ideal career, and people who mean the most to me recognize them.

Every day puts me closer to my ideal career.

Every day, I grow closer to my objectives.

My ambitions are attainable.

I am deserving of the greatest in life.

I am capable of achieving whatever that is placed before me with hard work and devotion.

I am overjoyed and thrilled to have landed my dream job.

I am overjoyed to have finally landed my ideal job.

I am competent, clever, and gifted.

I am currently working at my ideal job.

I am overjoyed to have finally landed my ideal job.

I am confident in my abilities and capabilities.

I am certain.

I am worthy of my ideal job.

I have the ability to manifest my ideal job.

I'm doing everything I can to get the job of my dreams.

I take another step forward every day.

When the time comes to make a shift, the perfect job will find me.

I am entitled to the greatest employment possible.

I am grateful for the riches in my life.

I'm a success.

My employer and coworkers like me.

People value my viewpoint and seek my counsel.

I have the support of the entire cosmos.

I can do everything I set my mind to.

All of my efforts will be rewarded in the end.

My work ethic is exceptional.

I am a great and skilled individual.

There are many chances for me to achieve out there.

My abilities are valued and appreciated.

I am deserving of a fantastic career.

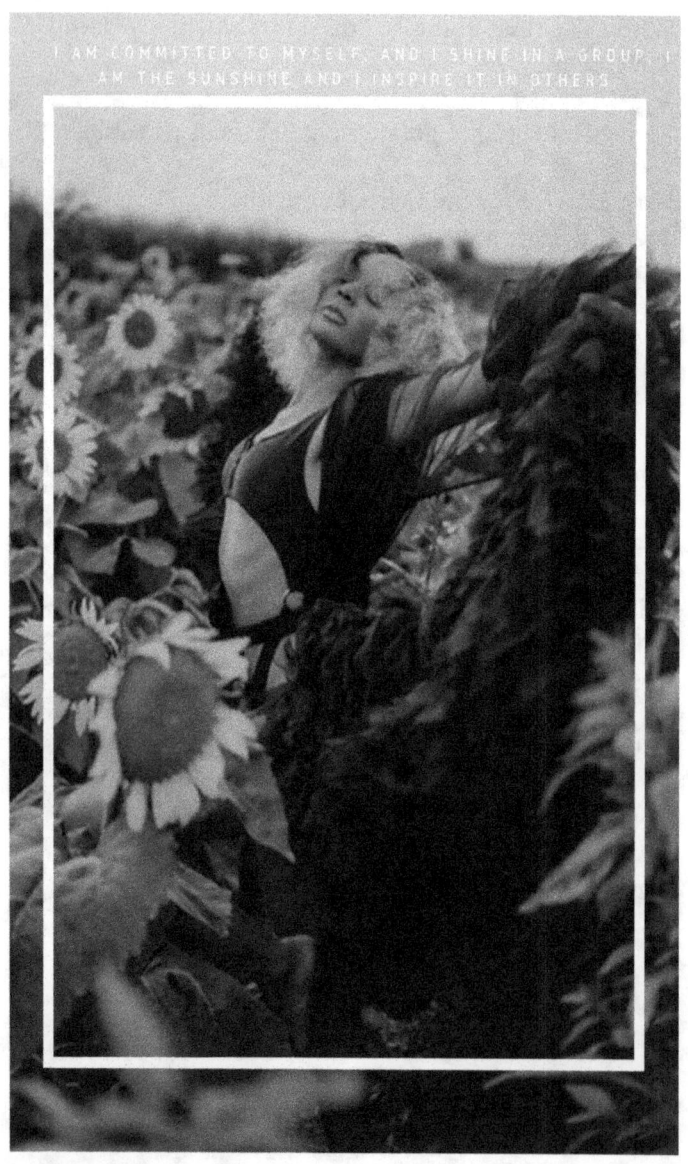

People who are aware of my talents trust me.

I possess the abilities to achieve where I want to go in life.

I have the qualifications to succeed in a job interview.

I am a responsible individual.

I'm visualizing my dream job joyously and joyfully.

I am qualified for any role.

My life improves every day, in every manner.

I will not settle for anything less than what I desire and deserve.

I was able to secure my ideal job.

It is safe to take risks since there is always a second opportunity if things do not work out the first time.

I really like working at my ideal job!

Affirmations When Looking For Work

I'm cool and collected.

I am capable of obtaining my ideal career.

I am upbeat and self-assured.

I am open to new possibilities.

I have the necessary knowledge and abilities for my ideal work.

I got the job of my dreams.

I am driven to discover my ideal work.

I seem to attract employment offers.

Job offers come to me with ease.

I am deserving of this position.

I am deserving of this position.

I thank the Universe for this chance.

I eagerly await good fortune and chances.

It is simple and thrilling to look for a new career.

There is a way where there is a will.

Affirmations for the Big Interview

I radiate self-assurance and confidence.

I'm quite good at job interviews.

I have excellent communication skills.

I talk with confidence and boldness.

My outstanding qualifications and talents will carry me through the job interview.

During job interviews, I feel at ease.

I have faith in myself.

I am a success magnet.

I am at ease, upbeat, and assured.

I thank the Universe for assisting me in obtaining this position.

I am really driven to succeed.

My enthusiasm is contagious. Job interviews come naturally to me.

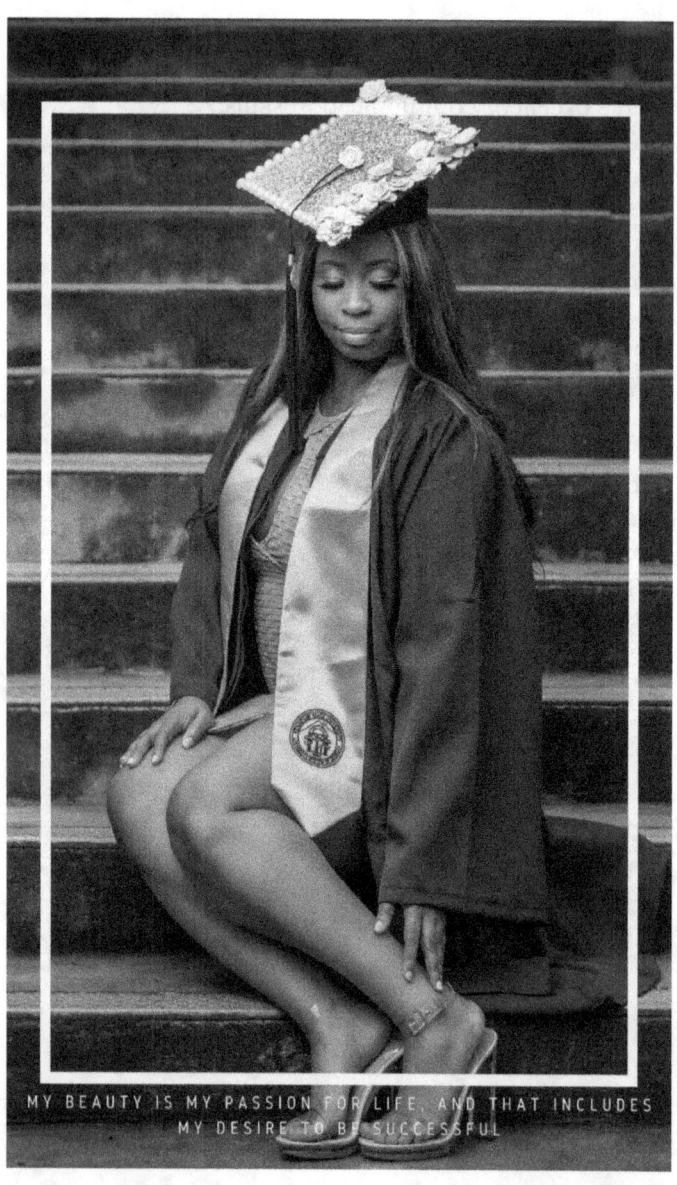

I'm really looking forward to starting my new work.

I stand out from the crowd. Interviewers are quickly impressed by me.

I am the ideal candidate for this job.

Affirmations for Your First Day at Work

I have the essential knowledge and abilities to execute the work successfully.

My employees are encouraging and supportive of me.

The job is enjoyable for me.

If I need assistance, I have it nearby.

My manager values my commitment and hard work.

I'm ready to start my new job.

I am adequately compensated for my earnest efforts.

I readily connect with my coworkers.

I like my profession and give it my all every day.

My new job makes me happy and fulfilled.

I can always get help and cooperation everywhere I go.

I look forward to going to work every day.

I am skilled at establishing interpersonal interactions.

I enjoy what I do.

Everyone at work admires me.

Affirmations to Keep You Motivated

I am confident in my own value.

My work is of high quality.

To be among the top, I must be talented and hardworking.

I put my all into whatever I do.

The outcomes I present are adequate confirmation of this.

I'm having the time of my life.

I am enthusiastic about what I do.

I let the Universe do its thing for me.

I have the fortitude to face my worries and anxieties.

I consider obstacles as chances to advance in my job.

I'm confident that the Universe has my back.

I am thankful for all of my blessings and triumphs in life.

I am filled with optimism, and this will result in wonderful consequences.

Affirmations to Succeed at Your Career

I am exactly where I want to be in my job.

I make good use of my time, skill, and energy in order to advance in my career.

I am driven and inspired to reach my professional objectives.

I give myself permission to advance in my job.

I provide myself permission to expand my knowledge and talents.

My moment has arrived and the sky is the limit for me.

I feel confident in my ability to achieve my job goals.

I control my own fate.

I deserve to advance in my career.

I have the knowledge and expertise to advance in my work.

Whatever I set my mind to, I can achieve.

I'm getting more and better opportunities.

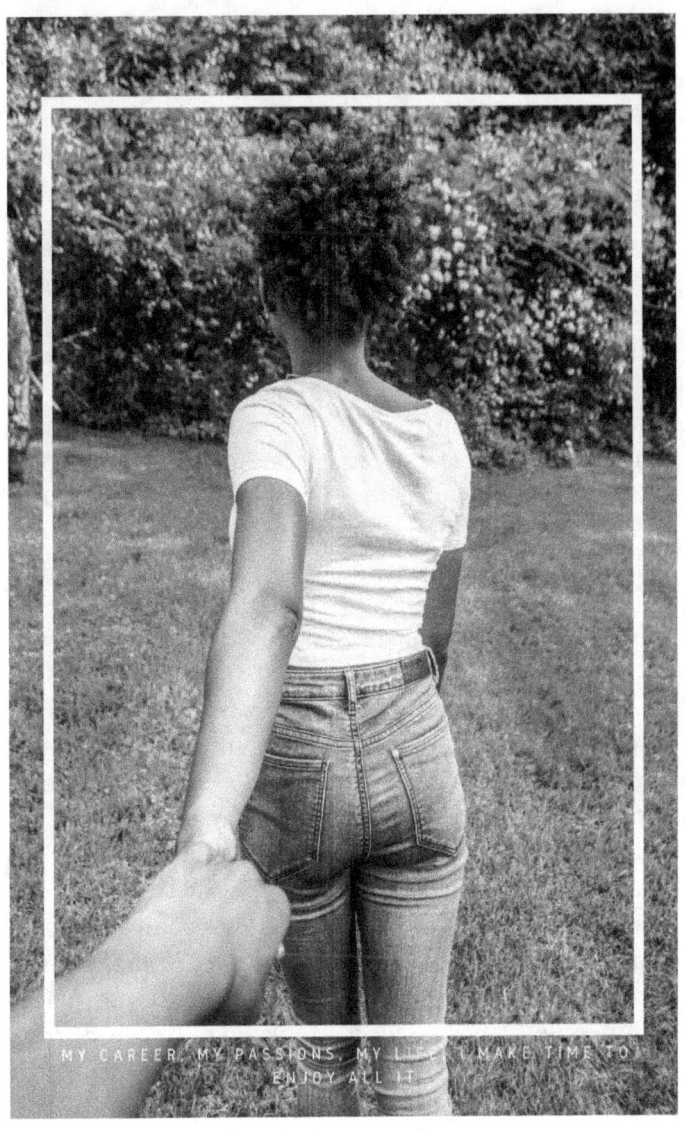

Conclusion

I hope that you have found all of the affirmations in this book pleasant to read. It may be hard to implement a schedule in the morning where you will include these affirmations so you can always try to do them during the day or at night. Many black women have the potential to be great in our present-day society, and sometimes you just need someone to help you realize that you have this potential. I hope this book has been successful in being that voice for you, the voice you will turn to when you are feeling unsure about your journey. With time, you will become the extraordinary woman that you envision yourself to be.

We all have dreams. Some of our dreams scare us so much we wouldn't dare pursue them. And sadly, sometimes we limit our potential because we don't think that we would be good enough for a dream we have for ourselves. I have seen this happen to countless women. A woman who grows up excelling in many fields but with a disadvantage of growing up in an impoverished neighborhood may feel some intense imposter syndrome when she has to approach places with people of her intellect. Books like this need to be placed at the forefront, to be the voices that such women will hear in their heads when they feel like giving up. Because if we are honest, life is not fair for such women. And yes, they may sometimes have to work a little harder than others to get where they need to go.

In the book we looked at three areas of concern where affirmations may be helpful. Firstly, we touched on welcoming the nature of mothers. We talked about how hard it can be for some black women to remain committed to their maternal instincts. So many of the black women in our communities are looking after children on their own. This means that they have to tend to things at home and maybe work to put food on the table as well. This is an exhausting task to place on one person's shoulders. But these women carry it in stride. I hope these affirmations will remind them of the power they have maternally, so that they can reconnect with the natural instincts they already have.

Secondly, we looked at affirmations that would seek to nurture the innocence of daughters. We spoke about situations where children would lose their innocence. Perhaps you can think of many other ways in which little black girls can lose their innocence. As a mother, you can choose to purchase this book for yourself and read that portion to your daughter. The two of you can have a bedtime routine where you would read a few of your favorite affirmations and discuss the events of the day in detail. They way mothers and daughters should.

Lastly, we looked at affirmations to manifest career dreams. These are generally for any black woman who wants to move forward in their life. They are for women in corporate careers, and even business careers.

Drop the Excuses—Dream Big, Think Positively, Live a Life of Accomplishment and Achievement

Introduction

Her skin reflects the sun, her hair defies gravity, and she shines with the luminosity of a million stars. Behold: the black woman. Yet, despite our ethereal grace we are often not treated the way we should be. Black women are treated as a minority, at times less than human. We have been belittled and pushed into a corner for far too long. All these years of suppression have made us want to dim our light, to stay unseen—hidden—in the corner, the world forced us into.

The world judges us relentlessly without even getting to know us. They see us as "too loud," they tell us to straighten our hair with chemicals, they hypersexualize us, and in the end, they mold us according to what they see fit. Yet that is not what black women are. We are more than the fabricated stereotypes which they claim us to be.

As black women, we do not need to hide in a corner anymore. We have every right to emerge from the dark space they put us in; like a butterfly emerging from its cocoon, we will also come forward with our wings spread and ready to take flight. Our wings are bold and brilliant in color, just like the rest of our bodies.

"You are altogether beautiful, my love; there is no flaw in you." (English Standard Version Bible, n.d., Song of Solomon 4:7)

The world will see black women for what we truly are. We are human and magnificent in our own way, just like anyone else. There is nothing wrong with how loud or quiet we may be; our tightly coiled hair is beautiful as it is; we are works of art and deserve to be appreciated and marveled at. We can be whoever and whatever we strive to be.

I have seen the struggles black women have had to endure. I, myself, have gone through them and so has my mother, my grandmother, and all those before her. The prejudice against our kind has gone on for too long, but not anymore.

My fellow black women, it is time for us to rise above our circumstances, and the best way for us to do that is by uplifting ourselves, as well as each other. We cannot afford to stay down forever—our ancestors did not endure so much for us to stay suffering. We have the ability within us to heal, and turn our pain into something useful, as well as something

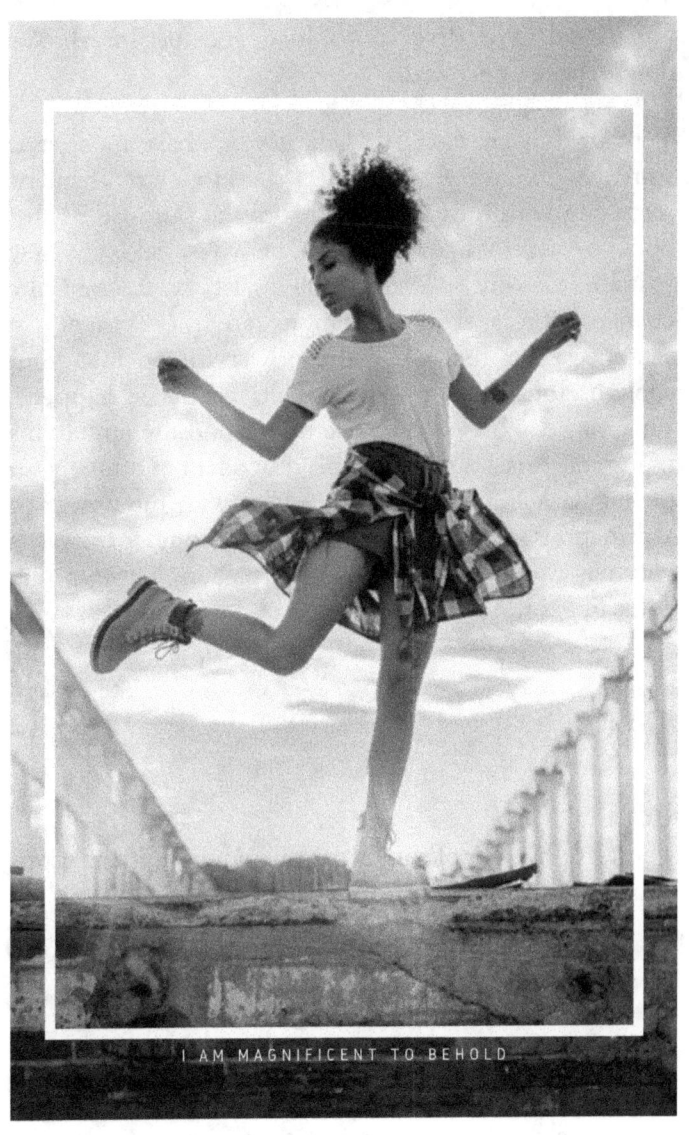

intentional. We deserve to love and be loved. We deserve to be nurtured.

Yet our journey into our new life or phase must start somewhere, and what better way to start than by searching within ourselves. That is the purpose of this book of affirmations—it is to help you adopt a new attitude to your life that will assist in creating the changes you seek. Affirmations are more than just sentences, for they have the power to tap into your subconscious, which is where all the magic happens. This magic allows you to rise up beyond the limitations the world sets for you as a black woman and take your power back into your hands. Along with the power of affirmations, there are also precious stones or crystals you may use to elevate and amplify your energy so that you can get the best results.

Goals

There are five simple goals for this book of affirmations which are as follows:

1. boosting black women's confidence in themselves

2. making black women realize that they deserve to live fulfilling lives

3. helping black women to set goals for themselves and accomplish them

4. instilling positivity
5. allowing black women to realize that they are not alone in their struggles

I am responsible for my own happiness and glorious destiny as a black woman. I have the power within me to mold my desires from dreams to reality. There is no right or wrong way to get this done, but I know I am more than capable. I allow my inner wisdom to guide me through the journey of life, and I have nothing to fear, for I am divinely guided and protected at all times.

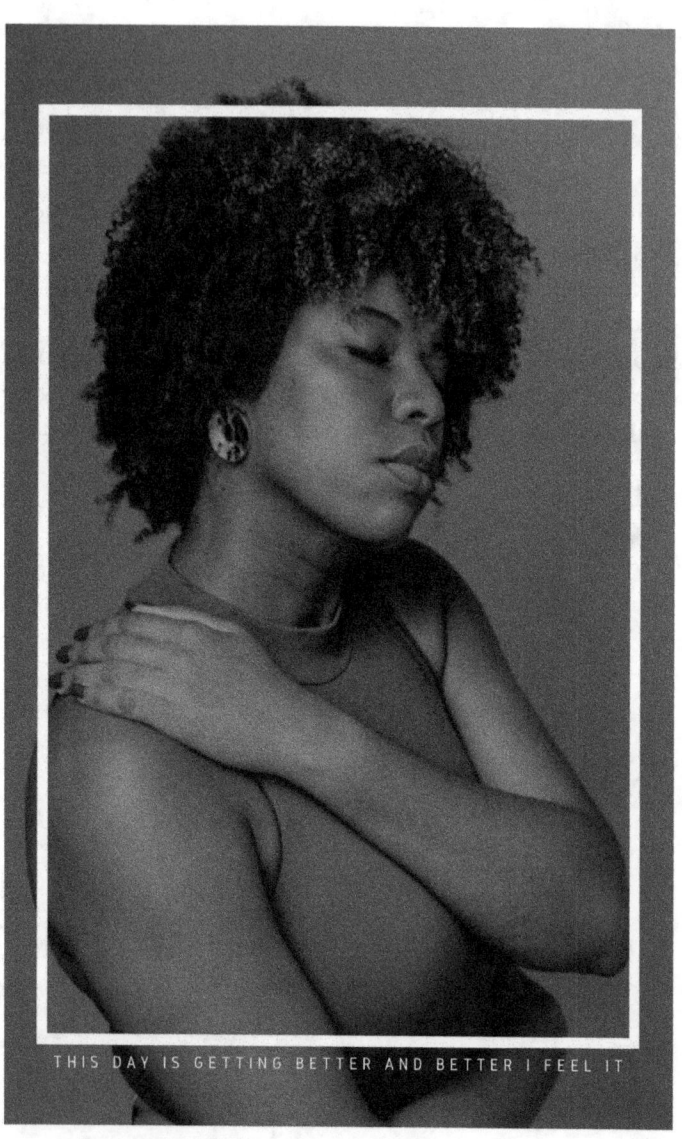

Chapter 13:

Drop the Excuses—Dream Big

Everything that I need to prosper is already within me, along with divine grace. But there are times when wanting to achieve big things is scary; we all feel afraid from time to time; it is a normal human emotion. Setting up aspirations can seem intimidating because we do not always know if they will work out in the end. These things have happened to me many times in my life, but the truth is you cannot allow fear to rule your life. As much as fear of things not working out is a natural response to the unknown, so is having goals. Setting goals, whether big or small, gives meaning to life. It is even better when a goal we set comes to fruition; it makes us feel good and makes the process worthwhile.

In this society, we black women are often belittled and feel discouraged when it comes to achieving our ambitions. Our ambitions can range from multiple things to wanting to get into a top college or university, starting a business, having a blooming love life, to making enough money to become financially stable.

Not every black woman is the same, and neither are our goals, but we have all had similar struggles when it comes to finding our place in society and overcoming stereotypes.

That is why we must find the light within ourselves. A light that ignites motivation within us. The recommended crystals for this chapter about dreaming big are Labradorite, Red Jasper, and Tiger's Eye. Labradorite assists in helping you find your purpose and provides clarity via inner wisdom; Red Jasper is for grounding yet will also improve your stamina to get going; Tiger's Eye increases motivation while also being a protective stone. Altogether these crystals will give you the burst of energy and motivation you need to achieve your goals.

"I can do all things through him who strengthens me."

—Philippians 4:13

Whether you will be listening to these affirmations or reading them, keep in mind to take them as if they were your own words. Listen or say each word with intention. Feel your soul being renewed by a positive change. My sister, you are the master of your own reality, and therefore you have what it takes to make your life beautiful and fulfilling. Step into your power as you say these words.

I allow myself to be a dreamer.

I am a creative individual; my creative energy is abundant, flowing through me like water from a river that never dries out.

I make goals for myself.

Even just setting out my goals is a brave thing to do, and I am proud of myself for that.

If my plan does not work out on the first try, I can always try again.

I do not fail—I simply learn, which helps me find a new path to achieve my goals.

I am a master manifester, and what is for me will never miss me.

I have what it takes to make it.

All that I desire is already within my grasp.

My goals and dreams are never too small.

I am passionate about the things I want to achieve; my passion is what drives me forward.

I am a successful black woman.

Big dreams are inspiring, but it is also okay to take baby steps.

The universe opens good doors for me.

My heart is open to receiving the fruits of my labor.

I clap for those who achieve their dreams before me—I know that my time to celebrate will come too.

I trust divine timing when it comes to my goals.

Obstacles are nothing I need to be worried about.

I accept congratulations and other prizes from those who have witnessed my achievements.

I remain humble and grateful for my successes.

I support my fellow sisters in reaching their dreams; I help where I can.

I effortlessly attract all that I desire.

Improvements are made everyday to make sure I meet my objectives.

I surround myself with like-minded people, those who understand me.

There is no such thing as failure; it does not exist in my vocabulary.

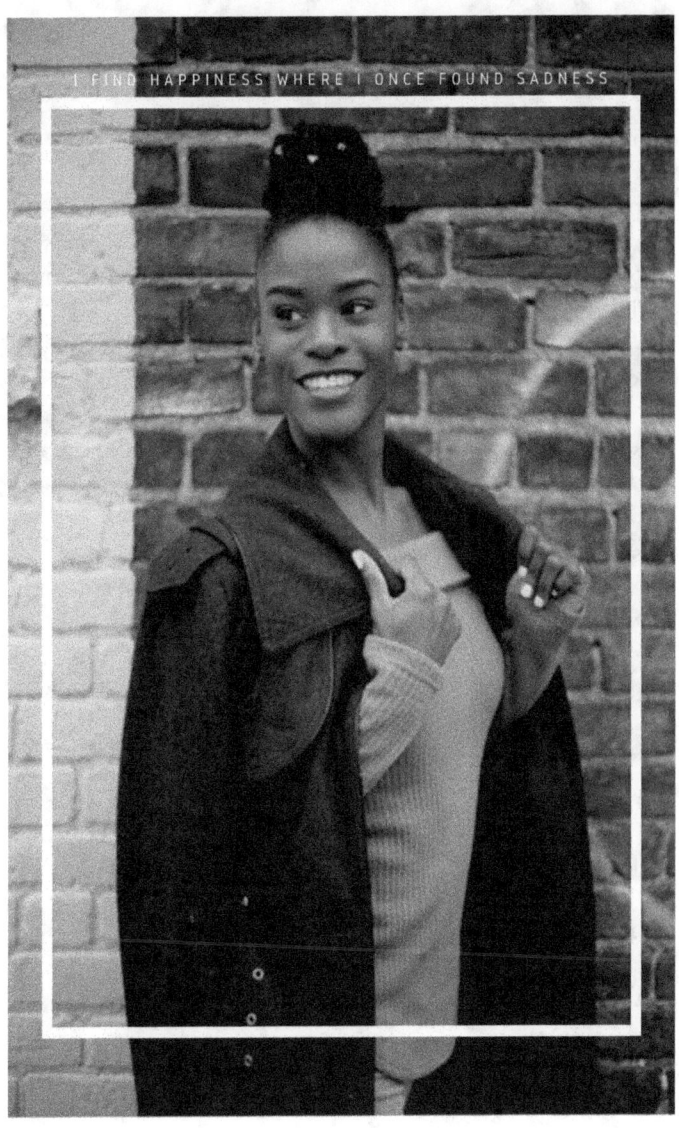

I have utmost faith in myself—I have what it takes to make it.

Fear of failure has no power over me.

I am divinely supported and guided.

My vision is crystal clear—I know what I want, and I make plans to get it.

The universe is abundant, and my success is unlimited.

The world and the opinions of other people do not determine my success.

I deserve to pay attention to my aspirations.

I physically write down my goals and how I plan to achieve them step by step—this makes me feel organized.

My life is just as important as anything else.

My dreams are protected and backed up by divine forces.

If others before me can do it, so can I.

I talk to God about my dreams, and He always listens.

My dreams do not have to be limited to being sky-high; they can go beyond space.

As a black woman, I will not settle for less because I know that I always deserve more.

I work hard to achieve my goals, while also taking the time to rest when needed.

I am strong-willed and determined.

I refuse to give up no matter how many times I stumble.

I will succeed despite what others say, even if they say I cannot succeed.

I make myself so proud.

Greatness is in my name; it is who I am.

Nothing and no one can stop me.

I am exceptionally talented.

I am good enough, in fact, more than enough.

The road to achieving my goals is a journey that I will happily embark on.

I respect that everyone's pathway to accomplishing their goals is unique—some may get there quickly while others take their time, and that is completely okay.

I will finish the things I start.

There is no such thing as losing in my eyes.

I learn new ways every day, which I can use to my advantage.

I refuse to hold doubt in my heart when it comes to my achievements.

I trust that it will all work out the way it is meant to, for my highest good.

Baby steps are just as valid as huge leaps; I will do whichever I am comfortable with.

I support my fellow black sisters in achieving their goals.

I take the time to celebrate my achievements without needing validation from others.

Challenges are seen as an opportunity to learn something new, and for growth in my eyes.

Setbacks do not phase me—I take the time to rest then I bounce back when I am ready.

I embrace my time to shine, and I will do so brightly.

I propel forward without fear.

There are many ways in which I can achieve my goals.

There is nothing wrong with asking for a helping hand—I have support from loved ones when I need it.

I use my gifts for good, and to help others.

I can and I will; there is no further excuse.

I quit making excuses or using habits like procrastination to avoid doing something.

I will not allow anything or anyone to hinder me.

I keep my eyes on the prize at all times.

I am enthusiastic about the work that I do.

I am in love with the journey that it takes to accomplish my goals; the end result will definitely be worth it.

I use different methods to motivate myself so that I can keep going.

Being productive, while striving for what I want to achieve makes me happy.

I FIND PEACEFUL MOMENTS TO MYSELF SOMETIMES

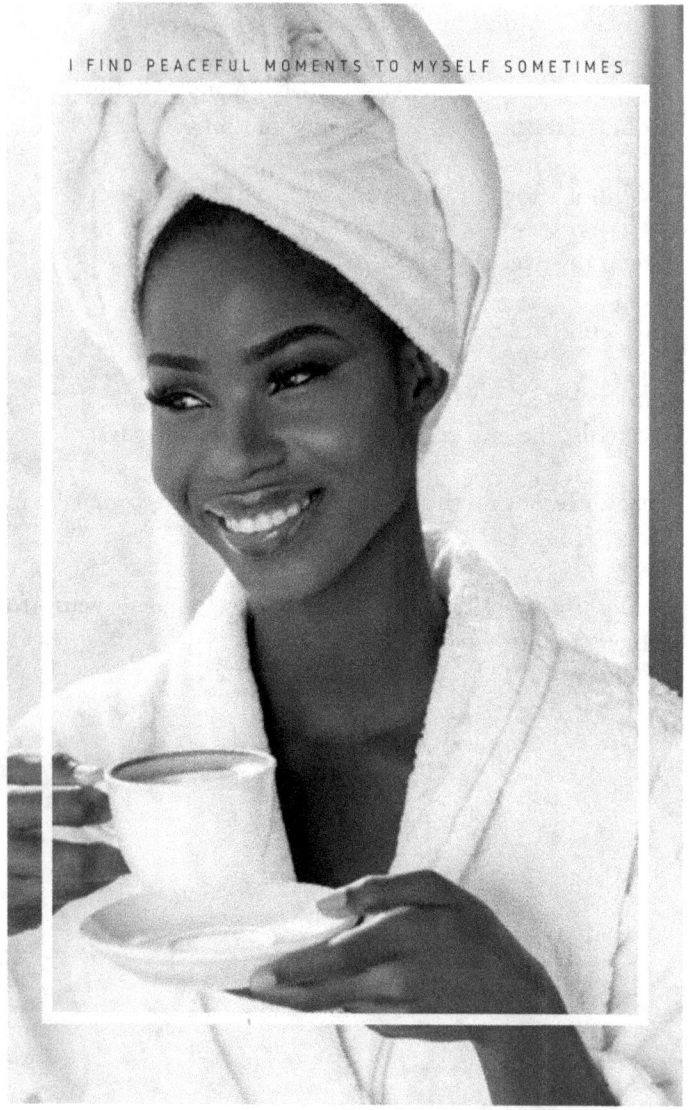

Victory always finds me no matter what the circumstances.

I am crowned for greatness; I will not stoop low for the sake of settling.

The universe is working in my favor and removing all obstacles out of my path.

I am doing the things I love with a fiery passion.

Resting is an essential part of working.

I can still make progress and grow even when I am taking a break.

I deserve a seat at the table with other achievers and successful people.

I am in this world to make a change, and I plan to make that a good change.

I never back down from a chance to learn something new.

I will not just try—I will do it, and I will do it well.

The sentence "I cannot" does not exist in my vocabulary.

I can do everything I set my mind to and I can do it a billion times over because I am determined.

There is no such thing as losing, only learning.

I am courageous in my pursuits.

The color of my skin has no impact on my success, and even if it does it still makes me a successful black woman who achieves greatness.

I am a conqueror.

My dreams are never too big; they are all capable of being achieved by me.

I am an ambitious black woman.

I work hard and play hard; I enjoy both to the fullest.

I have a healthy work ethic.

Chapter 14:

Think Positively

Being positive in this day and age is so important, especially when the world just seems to be going through so much havoc. What we consume and put into our minds is a lot like planting a seed. If you plant a bad seed, the sad will grow to reap bad fruit, yet if you plant a good seed then you will bear good fruit. Therefore, it is important to put good things into your mind. According to statistics, incorporating positive thinking into your life helps to alleviate depression, therefore making it beneficial to your psychological well-being. Of course, the body is nothing without the mind; the two are interconnected, along with your spirit.

"Whatever is true, whatever is honorable, whatever is just, whatever is pure, whatever is lovely, whatever is commendable, if there is any excellence, if there is anything worthy of praise, think about these things."

–Philippians 4:8

There are many ways to practice positivity, and it can be found anywhere if you are looking in the right places. Positive thinking can also be evoked through the Word, meditation, journaling, and also self-reflection. But at the same time, positive thinking does not mean that you must be completely oblivious to negativity and take issues lightly; instead, positive thinking simply encourages you to gain a new perspective on the things in your life, and ultimately the world around you. It also helps you solve problems and make decisions in a healthier manner since you will be calmer and will therefore be able to think clearly. Positive thinking can also be seen as something like a useful skill to have, especially when the going gets tough.

The crystals you can use for this chapter are Rose Quartz, Turquoise, and Clear Quartz. Rose Quartz is a love crystal and not just romantic love but also love between other people in your life and within yourself. Therefore, it is perfect for instilling positivity within yourself. Turquoise brings about peaceful feelings, and if you're someone who deals with social anxiety, it is also perfect for making you feel at ease in social situations, thus making it easier to spend time with others. Clear Quartz is the jack of trades in the crystal world, meaning it can be used for a variety of things, including absorbing negative energy in your surroundings and transmitting it into positive energy. This trio of crystals will help you in gaining a fresh, optimistic view of things.

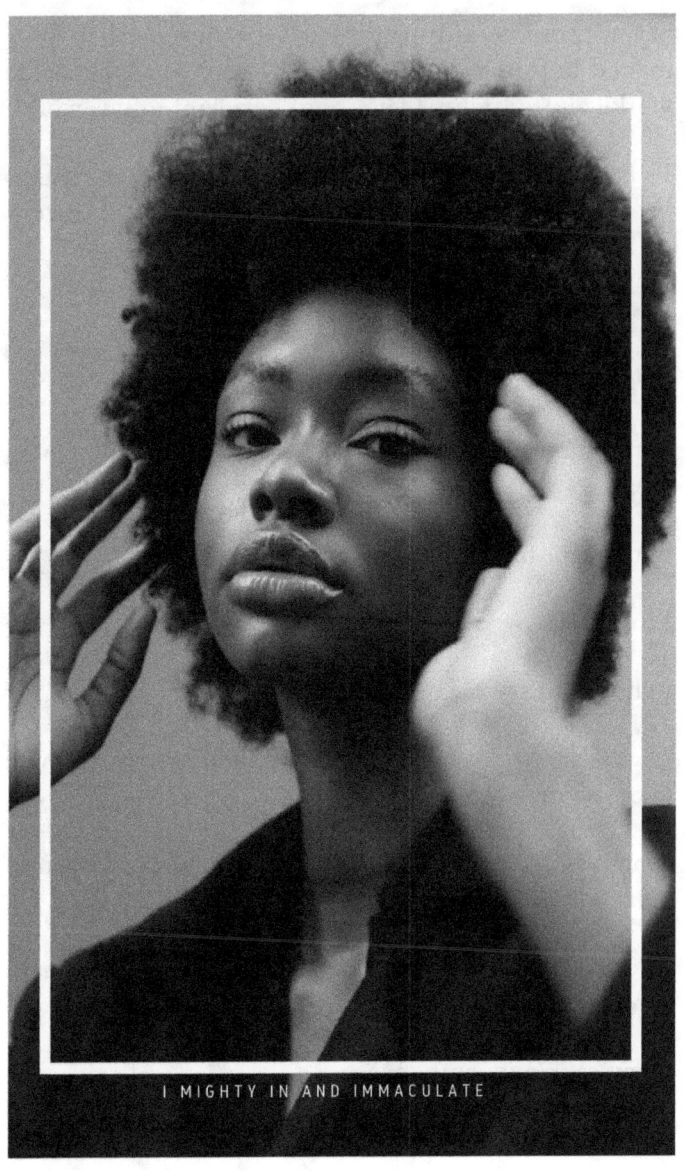

Saying positive affirmations will be beneficial to your mental health and will change the way you look at the world, and your life. I choose to be a light to this world.

I choose to love myself through all my shortcomings because I am human at the end of the day, and there is no need for me to be perfect.

I will uplift others in the best way I can.

Negativity has no place in my heart, mind, and soul.

My existence in this world will bring about something great.

I am beautiful in my own majestic way.

I love both myself and others.

I choose to see the good in others.

Each day I wake up with the feeling that something good is going to happen.

I express gratitude for all that I have, and I am open to gracefully receiving more.

Even on days when I do not feel so good, I will make sure I take good care of myself.

I stay calm and confident.

Kindness radiates through me.

My intentions are always pure and of the best intent.

I can still be strong yet soft, and vulnerable.

Even simple things can make me feel happy.

My joy comes from within me; it is not rooted in materialism and others' attention.

I am a blessing to those around me, as well as my community.

I am always doing my best.

I am a light to my fellow black sisters.

I am enveloped by positive energy—this energy can be felt by those around me.

I am kind to myself and others.

I am a caring and warm soul.

I am healing from the things that have hurt me in the past; I am in a safer space to heal now.

I am a magnet to miracles.

I surround myself with people who make me feel good about myself.

I am an optimist—even when it rains, I will come out with my own sunshine.

I will not be harsh on myself; instead, I will be patient with myself.

I make choices with good intentions, not only for myself but for other people too.

I find joy in lighting up someone else's day.

I hold sincerity towards other people.

Every storm will eventually pass, and the sun will beam again.

I possess a spirit of love; I do not harbor fear.

I have a clean conscience.

I know that I am loved beyond measure.

I refuse to hold onto grudges—I effortlessly let go of those who have wronged me so that I may have peace within.

I praise myself.

There is always a solution to a problem.

I have inner peace which has a positive impact on the world around me.

I am a reliable person.

My heart is always open to giving and receiving love.

I am an easy-going person—others find it easy to confide in me.

When I look in the mirror, I look at myself with admiration and think encouraging thoughts towards myself.

I am an avid spreader of joy.

I am the physical embodiment of love.

I do not mind being of service to others when they need my help, in fact, I take pride in helping others, knowing that I am making a positive impact in their lives.

I speak highly of others even when they are not around.

I treat others how I would want to be treated, which is with respect, humility, and compassion.

I accept others as they are.

BEING A SISTER IS MIGHTY TOO

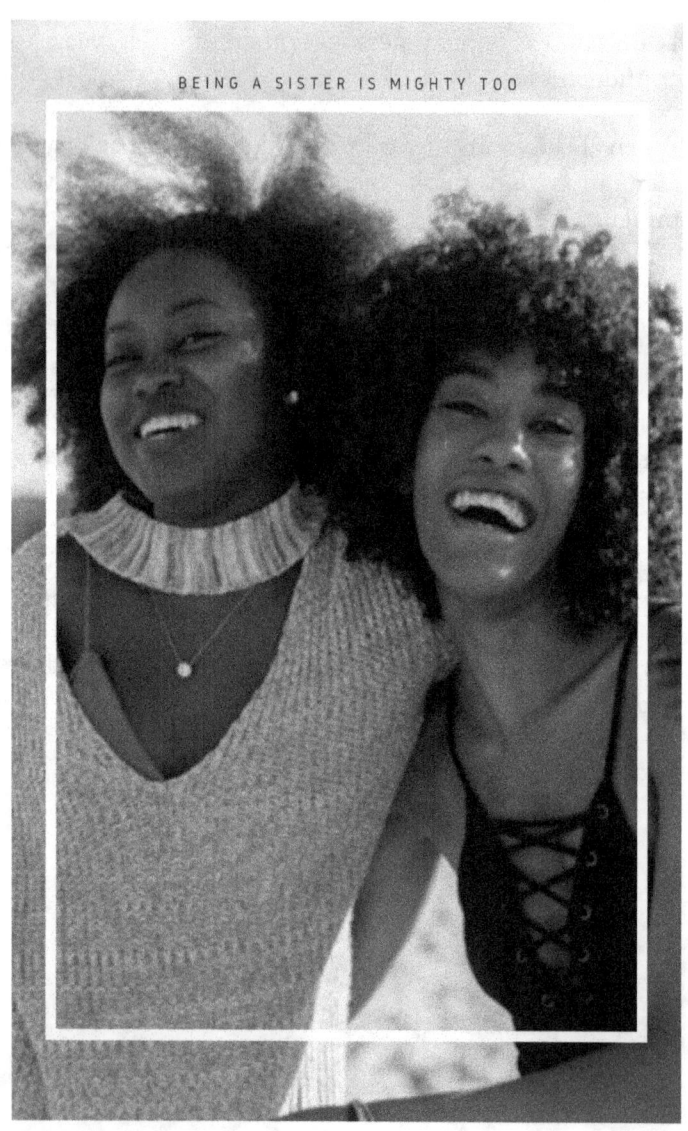

I understand that it is okay to not feel happy all the time, but I can see the good in every situation at the end.

I am helpful to my friends and family; I am a blessing to them.

Both my body and my mind are relaxed.

I choose to be peaceful even if the world wants the opposite reaction from me.

I will not stress about small things that have no relevance in my life.

My good thoughts radiate through me like sunlight.

I am above negative thoughts such as doubt, fear, and harsh self-criticism—the same goes for negative actions.

I choose to be a good person; through me, people will see that there is indeed love in this world.

I am a powerhouse for good vibes.

I release the things that no longer serve me—all of which are toxic and unhealthy and replace them with things that are way better.

People are comfortable being in my presence.

Chapter 15:

Live a Life of Accomplishment and Achievement

Setting goals and making plans to achieve them makes us feel like we have a purpose in this world, no matter how big or small these goals are. Although we may not always see it, even our mere existence on this planet has an impact. My melanated skin and eccentric hair are what make me special as a black woman, but it is not just about my appearance. I am brilliant in other ways too. I am intelligent and compassionate, and I persevere no matter how tough the going gets.

Just like anyone else, we black women have a lot to offer, and we should not let those who do not know any better belittle us. We deserve to be ambitious and reach for the stars. There is no need for us to struggle in life when there is no need to. Sure, we may not be as privileged as other groups of people, yet that does not mean we should stay down in the dumps and become victims of our circumstances. There is so much more to life than grappling from day to day.

"I came that they may have life and have it abundantly."

—John 10:10

The ideal crystals to use for this third chapter are Black Tourmaline, Citrine, and Blue Lace Agate. Black Tourmaline aids in boosting your morale after you have been in a tough place; to feel more confident, disciplined and for stepping into your true power use Citrine, as well as curbing depression and fear; Blue Lace Agate is the perfect healing stone for helping you step into your purpose and develop the courage to be who you want to be. Combined, these three crystals will help you take control of your life and achievements with newfound confidence and optimism. You are bound to be unstoppable.

My fellow black sisters, it is time we put a stop to the glamorization of our struggles. We deserve to live peaceful lives where we can be who we want to be. We deserve romantic relationships with partners who love us, and take care of us. We deserve to graduate and work at our dream jobs. We deserve to be financially secure. We deserve to live our best lives!

I am exceptionally talented and brilliant.

Good ideas come to me often.

I understand that life is a journey and I learn along the way.

I will not compare my journey to someone else's—everyone's experience on this Earth is unique.

I accomplish both big and small things in my life—all of which are equally important and deserve recognition.

My faith in the divine can move mountains.

Making mistakes is part of life; I will not let it hinder me from living a fulfilling life.

Every breath I take is testimony, and I celebrate that.

I am thankful for my life.

I am thankful for all my loved ones.

I forgive myself for past mistakes.

I choose to heal from the things that have hurt me in the past.

I am growing and blooming in my glorious purpose.

I live life boldly, and I am unapologetic about it.

I deserve the best of the best, the cream of the crop.

Instead of fretting about the past and stressing about the future, I focus on the present where all the magic is happening.

I share my love for others effortlessly.

I am living my absolute best life.

I consciously make good decisions in my life.

I am glad to have the opportunity to share my beautiful life with the beautiful people around me.

I have the potential to make a difference in this world.

This life is great and worth living.

My happiness is a top priority.

Me being here is a gift from God.

I live a life of unfathomable grace and favor.

I express gratitude daily; it forms part of my routine.

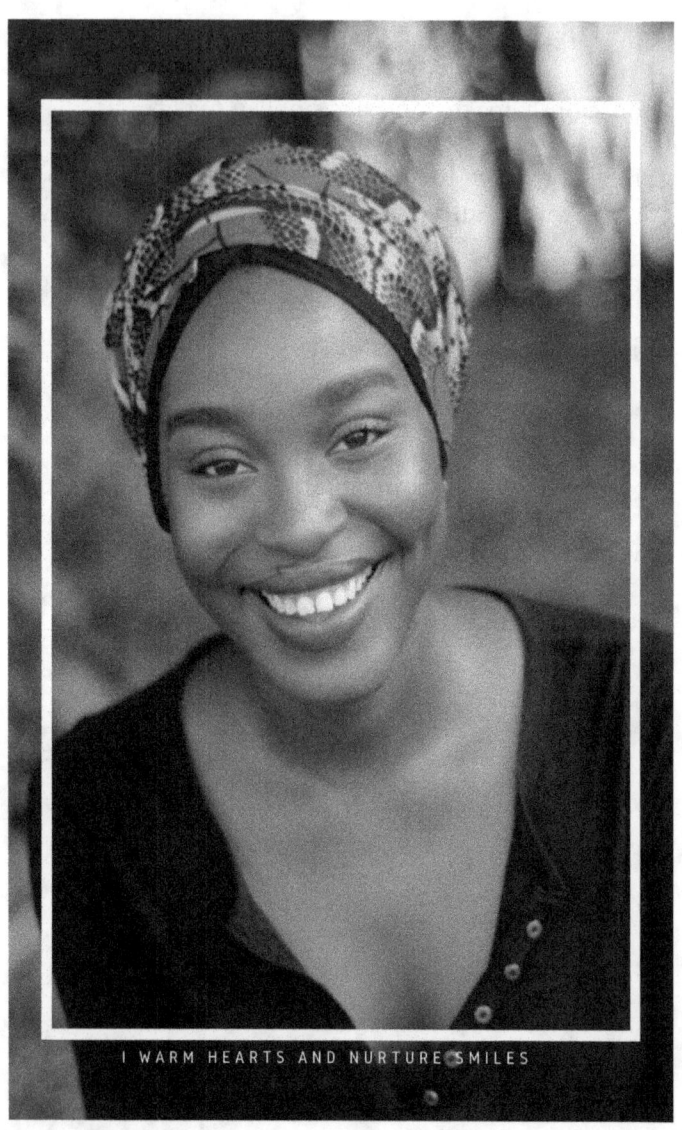

I WARM HEARTS AND NURTURE SMILES

Every single aspect of my life is flourishing—my finances, relationships, family, health, and spiritual wellbeing.

I set up the kind of structure I want in my life so that I can live happily according to my expectations.

The people I have in my life make me feel happy.

Although life may have its ups and downs, I will rise up at the end of the day.

I am constantly improving myself, and by becoming a better version of myself I can help others in return.

I am creating a beautiful life for myself.

I take the time to listen to my own intuition, which provides me with inner wisdom.

I deserve to live a soft life where I can freely nurture, and spoil myself.

I am worthy of all the finer things in life.

I deserve to enjoy this Earth that the divine created.

I am grounded in this present moment; I am stable and unshaken.

I may not always understand my family, but I have a deep love for them.

I appreciate my friends and family.

I am thankful for the lovely relationships I get to experience in this life.

I am an inspiration to others through all that I have achieved.

My aspirations are always valid.

Abundance is all around me, and I do not mind sharing this abundance with others since the supply will never run out.

I manifest the life that I want to live.

There is nothing wrong with wanting a luxurious and comfortable life.

Every day gets better and better.

Life is a journey, and I am enjoying every moment of it.

I handle my wealth with responsibility.

I am happy for others who are living their lives to the fullest.

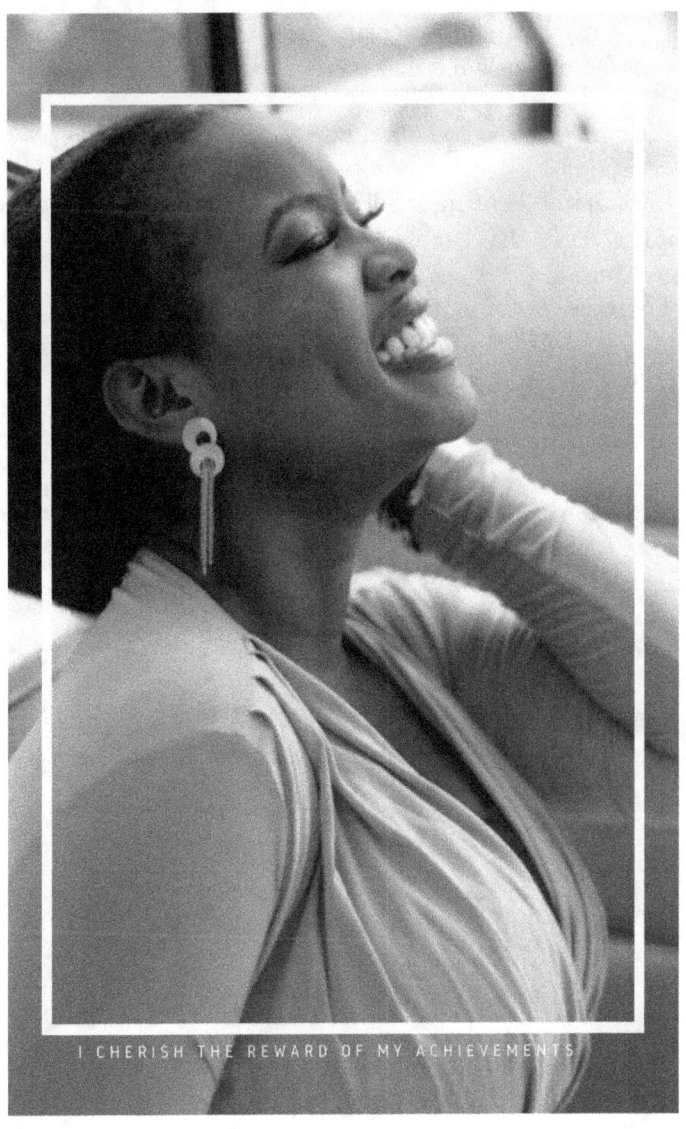

I CHERISH THE REWARD OF MY ACHIEVEMENTS

I live my life without shame or guilt for doing what is best for me, or what makes me happy.

I use my success to help others.

I am grateful for my body and all that it does for me—it is a vessel that enables me to get things done.

There is nothing wrong with wanting more out of life—I want big things, but that does not mean I do not take the time to appreciate the small things too.

I love my life.

I love the air I breathe.

I seek to have new experiences that will benefit me.

I am a valuable member in my community and the rest of society.

Great opportunities come my way frequently.

I will not compare my life to someone else's.

My friends and family may not share the same views of life as I do, but they support me, nonetheless.

I take charge as I am in control of my life.

There is no space in my life for others to bring me down or make me feel bad.

My relationships are strong and stand steady on solid foundations.

I know that my future is magnificent, and I can create it how I envision it every day.

I am a divine black woman.

I am worth it.

Every day is a great and blessed day.

I am grounded in my environment.

I am allowed to have pleasurable experiences.

My circumstances do not determine who I am, nor what I can do with my life.

Investing in myself is one of the best things I can do; I am the prize.

Various activities are incorporated into my day, which I enjoy.

I will not deny myself of luxuries; I have worked hard to deserve them.

It is okay for me to be figuring life out as I live it.

I am a powerful woman filled with a magnitude of love and strength.

I am worthy of everything that my heart desires.

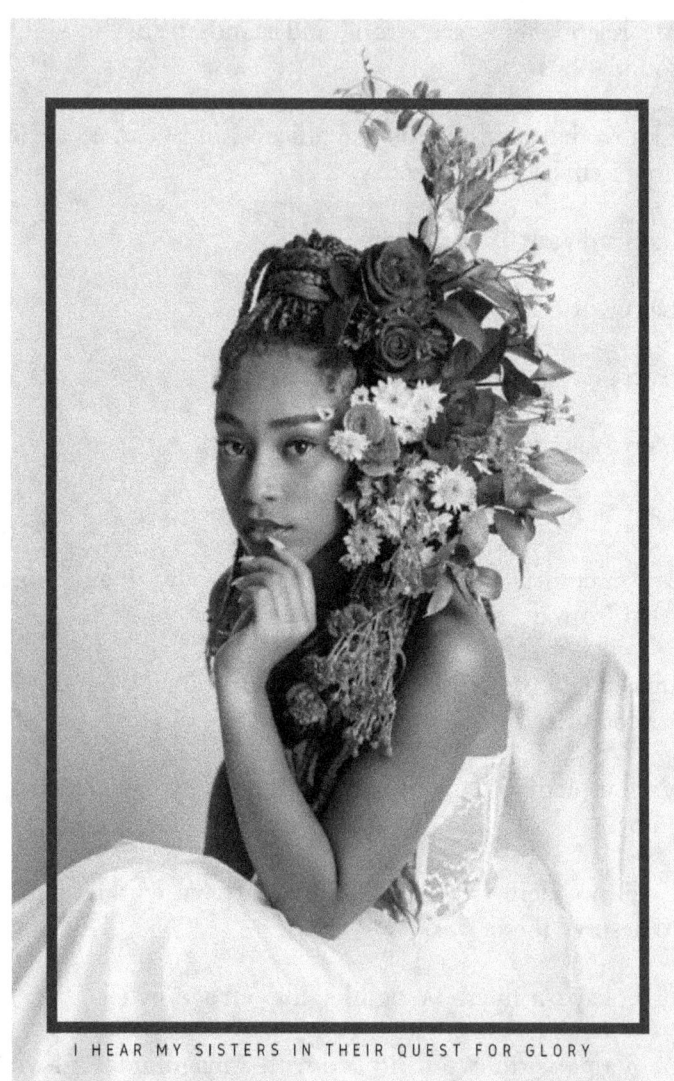

I HEAR MY SISTERS IN THEIR QUEST FOR GLORY

Conclusion

As a collective, black women all over the world have been through a struggle. A struggle for hope, love, power, and so much more. However, despite the recurring oppression, we have always persevered and fought against a world that has continuously prosecuted us. We only fight because we want our fair place in this world too. We also want to take walks without fear, wear whatever we want, plan our lives, be at peace, and above all, live happily.

Black women, you are perfect just as you are. There is nothing wrong with you, and you do not need to blend in or change yourself for the sake of fitting into this world. Instead, let the world see you as you are. Your light will never be too bright for the right people; if anything, they would love to see you shine.

There is no need for us to hold grudges against the world and its oppressors. The best thing for us as black women to do is to forgive them, and start healing ourselves from the inside out. We need to cater to ourselves so that we may improve, and do better. We are meant for nothing short of greatness. We deserve all the goodness.

This book of daily affirmations for black women is a start; with its recommendations of useful crystals, alongside the encouraging words from the Bible, you can finally start to spread your wings and take flight. You are beautiful, protected, and courageous. You have what it takes and even more, to achieve your dreams, have a positive mindset, and live the life which you desire. No matter how young or old you are, remember it is never too late to start.

"Trust in the Lord and do good; dwell in the land and befriend faithfulness. Delight yourself in the Lord, and he will give you the desires of your heart."

–Psalm 37:3-4

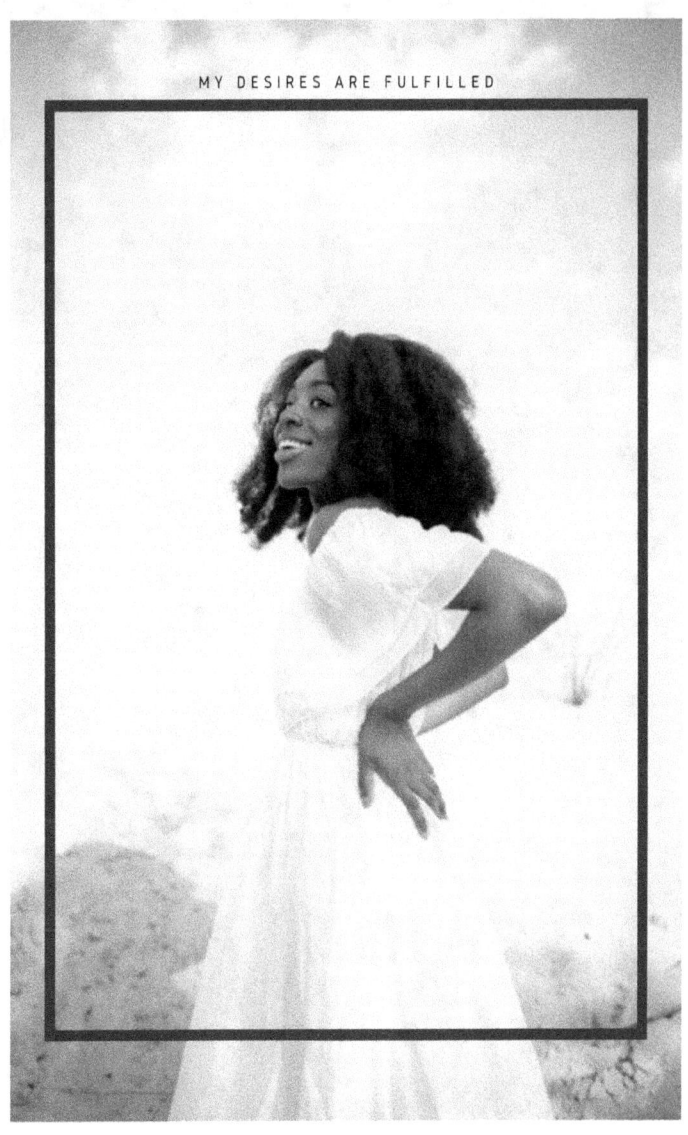

MY DESIRES ARE FULFILLED

References

Stone, Sharon (2022, February 14) Crystals And Healing Stones, Intuitive Way Publishing.

English Standard Version Bible. (n.d.). English Standard Version Online https://www.biblegateway.com/ (Original work published 2007)

35 Positive Affirmations for Black Women Around the World. (2020, February 19). Liveandearncanada.com. https://liveandearncanada.com/positive-affirmations-for-black-women/

Adigun, D. (2021, March 8). *Empowering Affirmations For Black Women By Black Women.* Wanderlust Calls. https://wanderlustcalls.com/empowering-affirmations-for-black-women-by-black-women/

Aggarwal, P. (2020, September 30). *Affirmations for the Divine Feminine.* Www.affirmation-Addict.com. https://www.affirmation-addict.com/blog/affirmations-for-the-divine-feminine?format=amp

Borge, J. (2021, May 19). *40 Positive Affirmations for a Sunnier Outlook*. Oprah Daily. https://www.oprahdaily.com/life/relationships-love/g25629970/positive-affirmations/

English Standard Version Bible. (n.d.). English Standard Version Online https://www.biblegateway.com/ (Original work published 2007)

Kristenson, S. (2021, November 20). *60 Affirmations for Inner Peace and Calm in Your Life*. Happier Human. https://www.happierhuman.com/affirmations-peace/

Wagner, K. D. (2016, February). *Connect with serenity. | Spirituality & Health*. Spirituality & Health. https://www.spiritualityhealth.com/articles/2016/02/01/12-affirmations-peace-and-calm

West, O. (2021, September 9). *100 Empowering Affirmations for Black Women Creators and Entrepreneurs*. Www.ourwestnest.com. https://www.ourwestnest.com/blogposts/2021/9/3/empowering-affirmations-for-black-women?format=amp

Diana, A. (2021, February 22). *30 Sex affirmations for A mind blowing sex life*. Ashley Diana.

https://ashleydiana.com/30-sex-affirmations-for-a-mind-blowing-sex-life/

Kristenson, S. (2021, December 6). *70 affirmations for self worth and love yourself More*. Happier Human. https://www.happierhuman.com/affirmations-self-worth/

Lerner, R., & Netlibrary, I. (1990). *Affirmations for the inner child*. Health Communications.

May. 19, E. S. |, & 2021. (2021, May 19). *100 positive affirmations for kids (and why they're so important)*. PureWow. https://www.purewow.com/family/affirmations-for-kids

Pathway2Success. (2018). *101 positive affirmations for kids- The pathway 2 success*. Thepathway2success.com. https://www.thepathway2success.com/101-positive-affirmations-for-kids/

Abundance No Limits. (2020). *75 New Job Affirmations For Manifesting Your Dream Job*. Abundance No Limits. https://www.abundancenolimits.com/new-job-affirmations/

Motivation Ping. (2019 February 26). *Inner Child Affirmations*. Motivation Ping.

https://motivationping.com/inner-child-affirmations/

Personal Creations. (2018 February 21). *52 Positive Affirmations to Inspire Moms + Printables.* Personal Creations Blog. https://www.personalcreations.com/blog/positive-affirmations-for-moms

Rotar, S. (2021 November 9). *45 Powerful Dream Job Affirmations - Mental Style Project.* Mental Style Project. https://mentalstyleproject.com/dream-job-affirmations/

Sasson, R. (2021 October 5). *40 Manifestation Affirmations for Love, Money and Dream Job.* Success Consciousness. https://www.successconsciousness.com/blog/affirmations/manifestation-affirmations/

Vidakovic, F. (2022 March 5). *50 Positive Affirmations For Women And Stressed Moms To Center You.* Inspiring Life for Moms and Kids. https://www.inspiringmomlife.com/positive-affirmations-for-women/

Bethesda Senior Living. (2020, July 21). *Bible verses that remind you to live a vibrant life.* www.bethesdaseniorliving.com. https://www.bethesdaseniorliving.com/blog/bi

ble-verses-that-remind-you-to-live-a-vibrant-life

Borge, J. (2021, May 19). *40 positive affirmations for a sunnier outlook*. Oprah Daily. https://www.oprahdaily.com/life/relationships-love/g25629970/positive-affirmations/

Collins, G. (2020, June 26). *85 powerful positive affirmations for living your best life | GIFT COLLINS*. Gift Collins. https://giftcollins.com/powerful-positive-affirmations-for-living-your-best-life/

Crawford, C. (2016, September 29). *10 crystals for positive energy & happiness*. lifehack. https://www.lifehack.org/469922/10-crystals-for-positive-energy-happiness

English Standard Version Bible. (n.d.). *English standard version online* https://www.biblegateway.com/ (Original work published 2007)

Grant, A. (2019, January 1). *365 positive affirmations to keep you going all year long.* Famous Ashley Grant. https://www.famousashleygrant.com/365-positive-affirmations/

Healey, J. (2018, January 15). *30 short daily affirmations for living your best life*. Healing Brave. https://healingbrave.com/blogs/all/short-daily-affirmations-for-living-your-best-life

Keithley, Z. (2021, October 4). *45 goal affirmations for achieving your dreams.* Zanna Keithley. https://zannakeithley.com/goal-affirmations/

Kristenson, S. (2021, December 12). *31 affirmations for positive thinking that will change your life.* Happier Human. https://www.happierhuman.com/affirmations-positive-thinking/

Rabea. (2018, September 15). *Affirmations for people with big dreams (+Freebie).* Rayowag. https://www.rayowag.com/affirmations-for-people-with-big-dreams/

St-Pierre, A. (2018, January 31). *Crystals and gemstones for achieving goals.* Liberate Your True Self. https://liberateyourtrueself.com/crystals-gemstones/crystals-gemstones-for-achieving-goals/

Tse, C. (2021, November 12). *18 energy crystals that might just change your life.* Slice. https://www.slice.ca/18-energy-crystals-that-might-just-change-your-life/

West, O. (2021, September 9). *100 empowering affirmations for black women creators and entrepreneurs.* Our West Nest. https://www.ourwestnest.com/blogposts/2021

/9/3/empowering-affirmations-for-black-women

Image References

Hezehiah, G. (2021, February 20) Photo by Gideon Hezekiah on UnSplash [image]. UnSplash.com. https://unsplash.com/photos/1I3_xTAXTxo

Emerson, B. (2019, June 18) Photo by Banjo Emerson Mathew on UnSplash [image]. UnSplash.com. https://unsplash.com/photos/9bu2Ujy-SsI

Masora, B. (2021, February 2) Photo by Ben Masora on UnSplash [image]. UnSplash.com. https://unsplash.com/photos/v2MkkWyASes

Irorere, D. (2021, April 21) Photo by Dennis Irorere on UnSplash [image]. UnSplash.com. https://unsplash.com/photos/ZDMms8xjS6Y

Darshan, D. (2017, November 15) Photo by Deva Darshan on UnSplash [image]. UnSplash.com. https://unsplash.com/photos/UtNLIFQT0dY

Hezehiah, G. (2021, July 30) Photo by Gideon Hezekiah on UnSplash [image]. UnSplash.com. https://unsplash.com/photos/57-0lgqwQOY

Gomes, J. (2021, February 3) Photo by Jeferson Gomes on UnSplash [image]. UnSplash.com. https://unsplash.com/photos/5BI8aExqwBo

Felicio, J. (2018, May 24) Photo by Jessica Felicio on UnSplash [image]. UnSplash.com. https://unsplash.com/photos/QS9ZX5UnS14

Felicio, J. (2018, November 27) Photo by Jessica Felicio on UnSplash [image]. UnSplash.com. https://unsplash.com/photos/lH973Qz0Iy4

Oyebanji, J. (2021, June 4) Photo by Joshua Oyebanji on UnSplash [image]. UnSplash.com. https://unsplash.com/photos/IxNjp3NprJw

Oyebanji, J. (2021, June 4) Photo by Joshua Oyebanji on UnSplash [image]. UnSplash.com. https://unsplash.com/photos/U86Zxi_Jer8

Omar, M. (2019, March 1) Photo by Mustafa Omar on UnSplash [image]. UnSplash.com. https://unsplash.com/photos/tEz8JU1j-00

Ankrah, M. (2021, March 2). *Photo by Melvin Ankrah on Unsplash* [Image]. Unsplash.com. https://unsplash.com/photos/PvzIJnfu1AU

David, J. (2019, August 16). *Photo by Jackson David on Unsplash* [Image]. Unsplash.com. https://unsplash.com/photos/BL_Q4zjduGU

Escrig, S. D. (2021, February 25). *Photo by Sergi Dolcet Escrig on Unsplash* [Image]. Unsplash.com. https://unsplash.com/photos/hrK7QVvOpH8

Fidele, E. (2018, September 3). *Photo by Etty Fidele on Unsplash* [Image]. Unsplash.com. https://unsplash.com/photos/nF8eo2nX374

Odunsi, O. (2019, January 13). *Photo by Oladimeji Odunsi Unsplash* [Image]. Unsplash.com. https://unsplash.com/photos/Wu3yqve2gnc

Graj, J. (2018, February 1). *Photo by Jernej Graj on Unsplash* [Image]. Unsplash.com. https://unsplash.com/photos/rlNibgIqi4o

Kiragu, I. (2018, June 17). *Photo by Ian Kiragu on Unsplash* [Image]. Unsplash.com. https://unsplash.com/photos/GSh_PwsZsPQ

Ma'aji, M. I. (2020, May 5). *Photo by Muhammadtaha Ibrahim Ma'aji on Unsplash* [Image]. Unsplash.com. https://unsplash.com/photos/anwtuO4gNqc

Odunsi, O. (2018, November 18). *Photo by Oladimeji Odunsi on Unsplash* [Image]. Unsplash.com. https://unsplash.com/photos/aU_eOcelLhQ

Yelizarov, V. (2021, April 4). *Photo by Vladimir Yelizarov on Unsplash* [Image]. Unsplash.com. https://unsplash.com/photos/tGRks1CV_HA

Aboh, S. (2020). Mother and Child. In *Unsplash*. https://unsplash.com/photos/RGomcmMkTEA

Assanne, G. (2020). Long Dress. In *Unsplash*. https://unsplash.com/photos/mJmxnpJTr8w

Effiong, D. (2021). Black and Green. In *Unsplash*. https://unsplash.com/photos/5ZrcEPi8ihE

Fellicio, J. (2018). Flower girl. In *Unsplash*. https://unsplash.com/photos/OoGcbDAsJ98

Kojo, N. (2020). Black and White. In *Unsplash*. https://unsplash.com/photos/I2JwX7RG8Cs

Odunsi, O. (2017). Blue. In *Unsplash*. https://unsplash.com/photos/hwsqCAHgqQM

Rikonavt. (2020). Black Hat. In *Unsplash*. https://unsplash.com/photos/jwkVc8Jw1Ck

Sikkema, K. (2019). Locs. In *Unsplash*. https://unsplash.com/photos/kT2VGgFXrAU

Von, M. (2020). Yellow. In *Unsplash*. https://unsplash.com/photos/BhcutpohYwg

Yaw-Otoo, N. (2021). Military Scarf. In *Unsplash*. https://unsplash.com/photos/x-S01itDdnk

Aboh, S. (2020). *Family* [Image]. Unsplash. https://unsplash.com/photos/S1NYr9djLtU

Christina. (2019). *Woman* [Image]. Unsplash. https://unsplash.com/photos/L85a1k-XqH8

Kombs, K. (2018). *With him in tow* [Image]. Unsplash. https://unsplash.com/photos/eDvztabelj8

Marquez, J. (2021). *Sunflower* [Image]. Unsplash. https://unsplash.com/photos/dXHD4FCi2ek

Masora, B. (2021). *People* [Image]. Unsplash. https://unsplash.com/photos/8hLjTQCNbNY

Nation, A. (2020). *Work* [Image]. Unsplash. https://unsplash.com/photos/vDxvAmuNDK8

Reis, J. (2020). *Relationships* [Image]. Unsplash. https://unsplash.com/photos/9ooYPL2Tffg

Rickerts, A. (2021). *Class of 2021* [Image]. Unsplash. https://unsplash.com/photos/QampqotXmGk

Vessels, Z. (2019). *Black Queen* [Image]. Unsplash. https://unsplash.com/photos/rWxMfj9y0F4

Virgin, I. (2018). *Ballerina* [Image]. Unsplash. https://unsplash.com/photos/Pb8_guWhws4

Akachi, P. (2018a, July 5). *Photo by Prince Akachi on Unsplash.* Unsplash.com. https://unsplash.com/photos/i2hoD-C2RUA

Akachi, P. (2018b, November 15). *Photo by Prince Akachi on Unsplash.* Unsplash.com. https://unsplash.com/photos/NcInpj4RFAM

Balla, J. (2021, July 9). *Photo by J. Balla Photography on Unsplash.* Unsplash.com. https://unsplash.com/photos/kChMFvup-0o

Chloe, A. (2017, December 9). *Photo by Alexis Chloe on Unsplash.* Unsplash.com. https://unsplash.com/photos/TYDkKEgc0Fg

Good Faces. (2021, September 27). *Photo by Good Faces on Unsplash.* Unsplash.com. https://unsplash.com/photos/62wQhEghaw0

Rosa, D. (2018, April 11). *Photo by Diego Rosa on Unsplash.* Unsplash.com. https://unsplash.com/photos/Yyk4OmVJAyE

Stupak, T. (2019, May 16). *Photo by Taisiia Stupak on Unsplash.* Unsplash.com. https://unsplash.com/photos/mt7BDYW0qLU

Thought Catalog. (2018, February 5). *Photo by Thought Catalog on Unsplash.* Unsplash.com. https://unsplash.com/photos/23KdVfc395A

Wade, T. (2021, April 15). *Photo by Troy Wade on Unsplash.* Unsplash.com. https://unsplash.com/photos/C0lEKXFUvmA

Yelizarov, V. (2021, January 1). *Photo by Vladimir Yelizarov on Unsplash.* Unsplash.com. https://unsplash.com/photos/crnAlC9fcqE

www.ingramcontent.com/pod-product-compliance
Lightning Source LLC
Chambersburg PA
CBHW070653120526
44590CB00013BA/944